IC Bladder Pain Syndrome

The Alternative Medical Treatment
for Interstitial Cystitis

∽

By Dr. Bill Dean

Dedication

This book is dedicated with all my heart to my loving wife, Diana, who has been a great teacher and supporter in my work. It is also dedicated to disease, for She becomes our greatest teacher on our journey to health.

Acknowledgments

Thanks to the many IC patients over my years of practice who have taught me so much about themselves and the imbalance that causes them pain.

Thanks to all my matter science healers and teachers who taught me about the science of healing in medicine and surgery.

Thanks to all my energy science healers and teachers:

Vasant Lad, BAMS, MASc

Deepak Chopra, MD

David Simon, MD

Foreword

Ayurveda is a timeless healing science, having its roots in Vedic literature, which is more than 5,000 years old. There is deep wisdom in the Sanskrit language. The ancient texts are written in a form of poetry called sutras. The Sanskrit word sutra means thread and it also means to suture. Just as pieces of cloth are sutured together to create a beautiful piece of the clothing, the poetry of sutras act as pneumonic devices to piece together quantities of knowledge. Instead of the digital recordings we use today to store texts, the ancients memorized this poetry. They learned these from their teacher or guru, who supplemented the knowledge of the sutras with further instruction.

The oldest authoritative text on Ayurveda is the *Charaka Samhita*. A classic sutra says that in Ayurveda there are three basic doshas: vata, pitta, kapha. These are the three organizations that govern the individual's unique psychophysiology and they are present in every RNA and DNA molecule as the genetic code of that person. This genetic code is called prakruti, the person's constitution. Due to changes that we all experience such as aging, changes in diet, in season, relationship, job, and environment, our prakruti dosha undergoes change as well. This resultant altered status of the doshas is called vikruti. Vikruti is not necessarily disease, but it creates the potential space in which this can happen.

The sutra continues with *dosha dushya samurchana janito vyadhi*. This says that every disorder or disease is simply aggravated dosha. One of the doshas leaves their own site and enters general circulation. It then lodges in a defective space in the body, called khavaigunya. This khavaigunya is a potential weakness or pre-pathological lesion. It could be anywhere in the body, such as in the lungs, bladder, kidneys, or heart. A potential weakness in an organ is usually from a genetic predisposition. Ayurveda says that we carry the cellular memory of our great-grandparent's illness. That memory may be stored within the DNA. From this cellular genetic memory, our bodies contain this potential weakness in the corresponding organ. For example, if one's grandfather died of a heart attack, that memory of a heart attack may be present within the connective tissue or muscles of the heart. As this person ages, s/he may have high blood pressure, cholesterol, or triglycerides, leading to heart disease or cardiac arrhythmia.

This can happen with any other disease. Cystitis is a condition of bladder inflammation that usually occurs because of excess pitta in the urinary passage. Ayurveda identifies some conditions as being inflammation without infection. Modern medicine used to say there was no fever without infection; fever was considered a sign of infection. Nevertheless, Ayurvedic texts say there is a possibility of fever without an infection, and now modern medicine has determined that there is pyrexia (fever) of unknown origin. Interstitial cystitis (IC) is a disorder where there is no bacterial involvement, no infection. Ayurveda says these functional changes in the kidneys, prostrate, bladder, and urethra are possible because of changes in the bodily doshas.

The Role of Vata Dosha in Inflammation

Vata is the principal of movement, and all involuntary movements are governed by vata dosha. Vata governs such things as peristaltic movement of the GI tract, movement of the cardiac muscle, subtle movement of the bronchial tube, and the movement of the bladder. Voluntary muscles circulation are governed by vyana vayu (circulatory movement), causing apana vayu (outward movement) and prana vayu (inward movement) to work with synchronicity and create proper action.[1] This synchronicity is shown in the smooth muscles of the bladder and the ureter, as well as the fine movements of the glomeruli and Bowman's capsule of the kidneys of the kidney.

If normal movement is delayed then there is stagnation. Vata is **dry, light, cold, mobile,** and **clear**. Because of the **dry** quality, there is **dryness** and this can create irritation and inflammation. If the **mobile** quality is diminished, there is a stagnation of excretory functions leading to congestion and inflammation. This inflammation is not necessarily from a bacterial or viral cause.

---

[1] The vayus are the five subdoshas of vata, each with a specific direction of movement in the body.

The Role of Pitta Dosha in Inflammation

Pitta dosha is **hot, sharp, penetrating, oily liquid,** and **sour**. When there sluggish movement within the wall of the bladder, pitta stagnates in the interstitial space of the bladder wall and because of its **hot** quality creates inflammation, the **sharp** quality creates irritation, and **sour** quality can cause acidic pH. This stagnant pitta within the interstitial spaces of the bladder causes a painful inflammatory bladder condition. Its etiology is unknown, but Ayurveda says it lies in a pitta-provoking diet, lifestyle, and emotional reactions.

In this book, Dr. Bill Dean elaborates on the history of IC as a chronic disease and any chronic condition is a direct result of long lingering dosha within the khavai-gunya. This defective space can be caused by a weakness in the tissue or organ. Ayurveda describes seven tissues (dhatus) that govern the building architecture of the various organs and systems of the body. If we take a section of the bladder, it has a mucous lining, which is rasa dhatu or plasma tissue. Underneath the mucous lining, there is a lining of capillaries, which is rakta dhatu, the blood tissue. Next is the lining of the muscle, which is mamsa dhatu. There may be a little adiposity within the two muscular layers to hold the muscle fibers together and that is meda dhatu. Outside is a serous layer, which contains the asthi and majja dhatus, the bone and nerve tissues. These seven dhatus are present throughout the body and they can be particularly present in every organ, including the gastrointestinal and respiratory tracts.

Interstitial cystitis is caused by vata pushing pitta into the bladder. Then within the interstitial space, pitta stagnates because of lack of movement. When there is inflammation, pain, and irritation, there is increased urination. This condition may occur because of exposure to certain drugs like ciprofloxacin or sulfonamides. These drugs have a bitter and pungent taste, which can increase pitta. Ayurveda teaches that substances can provoke the doshas because of their qualities, which will increase the like qualities of the dosha. Pitta provoking substances include sour foods, citrus fruits, and **hot** peppers. Similarly, some drugs may trigger pitta in the body. Increased pitta can lodge there into the interstitial space creating interstitial cystitis.

According to modern science, interstitial cystitis is most common from the age 30, which is the pitta time of life, according to Ayurveda. While not life threatening, the pain of IC can make the person's life intolerable. To avoid the pain of urination, the person may consume less quantity of fluids. Then they may retain urine and as a result, the urinary pH becomes acidic and then it becomes highly concentrated, causing further discomfort, irritation, and inflammation. This becomes a vicious cycle that negatively affects the individual.

This chronic condition is long lingering pitta dosha in the capillaries and muscle tissues of the bladder. It is a systemic disorder connected to the urinary tract, but it is a non-infectious, non-malignant condition. Dr. Bill Dean teaches us how to manage this uncomfortable disorder. His profound experience helps the person seek balance through proper diet and lifestyle in conjunction with Ayurvedic protocols for mind and body.

According to Ayurveda, there is a universal mind (vibhu) and individual mind (anu), and then there is cellular mind, a very subtle form of mind. Mind manifests even at the cellular level, and it has thoughts, feelings, and emotions because thinking is a natural, continuous function of the mind. Mind is judging and evaluating because that is the function of the mind. Ayurveda classifies the mind into these three major types: vata, pitta, and kapha types.

Fear, anxiety, insecurity, and loneliness are vata emotions. Anger, hate, envy, jealousy, and irritability are pitta emotions and attachment, greed, and possessiveness are kapha emotions. In general, people with IC have pitta predominant prakruti and pitta predominant vikruti.

The mind can also have pitta dosha predominant. Perfectionistic, hardworking people who are intensely goal-oriented can become irritable and upset with themselves when a goal is not achieved. These factors of the mind can trigger the pitta dosha, causing pitta to increase to the point that it enters into general circulation in the body.

This aggravated dosha circulating throughout the body is seeking a place to settle. The bladder may have a potential weakness from a previous infection or disease, from pregnancy, a pitta-provoking diet, relationship problems, or even from sex.

Unfortunately, one of the symptoms of IC is increased urination frequency that is accompanied by pain and irritation. There is no curative medical therapy. However, if we try to balance this complex network of the doshas, of vata pushing pitta into the bladder, we can resolve this condition. Dr. Dean has given a wonderful dietary program that will help this condition.

Aloe vera is a natural pitta-pacifying herb. It is anti-inflammatory and has a soothing, calming, cooling effect on the bladder wall. It helps to control urinary bladder inflammation. As the patient begins to benefit from the pitta-soothing diet, they should not be afraid to take in more liquid. They can start having liquids like water, coconut water, pomegranate, cranberry, or watermelon juice, or cucumber milk. Cucumber milk is quite pitta soothing for IC. Spices that can calm down pitta are cumin, coriander, and fennel. Cumin, coriander, fennel tea is quite effective in dealing with interstitial cystitis.

Energy stagnation in the mind and cravings can go together. Cravings can indicate a doshic imbalance or deficiency of certain elements. The body has its own intelligence. When pitta is high, a person naturally craves sweet, bitter, and astringent tastes, which act as cooling, calming, and soothing substances for pitta. That is a healthy response for the body. However, if there is long-standing doshic aggravation and agni is suppressed, the body builds ama. Ama is a toxic, morbid metabolic waste. Ama covers the cellular membrane and pervades the interstitial fluid, resulting in impaired cellular intelligence. Even though there is high pitta in the body, the person craves hot, spicy foods, which can further aggravate pitta. This is called perverted intelligence.

A clinician or physician can help to discover if this craving is natural and normal or unnatural and abnormal. Abnormal cravings are created by sama dosha – dosha with ama. Sama dosha creates perverted cravings, such as a kapha person wanting ice cream, yogurt, or other cooling foods.[2] It is beneficial to know whether a craving comes from the bodily intelligence or from doshic aggravation, so we can follow a proper diet and lifestyle.

Dr. Dean takes you through the patient's journey of dealing with IC and the situations that aggravate it. He then shows you new ways to think about this condition and to find balance. He takes you carefully through the dietary and herbal recommendations, followed by practices that support these lifestyles changes. This is a very practical guide for dealing with this problem on a day-to-day basis for those who have interstitial cystitis.

This book on IC is good news for all patients who suffer with the chronic pain of this disorder. It will definitely help to alleviate their suffering and make their lives happier, peaceful, and blissful. Dr. Bill has given a numerous practical guidelines regarding breathing exercises, meditation, yoga practice, oleation, herbal remedies,

---

[2] Kapha dosha shares similar qualities—heavy, slow, cold, dense—with these foods. Because of these shared qualities, these foods will tend to increase kapha dosha in the body.

and marma therapy that will assist in everyday comfort. I'm sure people will cherish this book throughout their lives.

Vasant Lad, B.A.M.&S., M.A.Sc.

Albuquerque, New Mexico

April 2013

For a New Beginning

In out-of-the-way places of the heart,
Where your thoughts never think to wander,
This beginning has been quietly forming,
Waiting until you were ready to emerge.
For a long time it has watched your desire,
Feeling the emptiness growing inside you,
Noticing how you willed yourself on,
Still unable to leave what you had outgrown.
It watched you play with the seduction of safety
And the gray promises that sameness whispered,
Heard the waves of turmoil rise and relent,
Wondered would you always live like this.
Then the delight, when your courage kindled,
And out you stepped onto new ground,
Your eyes young again with energy and dream,
A path of plenitude opening before you.
Though your destination is not yet clear
You can trust the promise of this opening;
Unfurl yourself into the grace of beginning
That is at one with your life's desire.
Awaken your spirit to adventure;
Hold nothing back, learn to find ease in risk;
Soon you will be home in a new rhythm,
For your soul senses the world that awaits you.

~ John O'Donohue ~

Table of Contents

Why I Wrote This Book

In my many years of practicing urology, I have seen a multitude of men, women, and children whose lives were affected by chronic interstitial cystitis (IC), non-bacterial cystitis, or chronic prostatitis. During this professional journey, my path crossed with Deepak Chopra and later Dr. Vasant Lad, who became my mentor and helped me glimpse the practice of classic Ayurveda, an energy science.

With personal application of these energy science practices, I saw my health begin to soar, so I decided to offer the healing techniques to my patients with difficult urological problems. I began seeing astonishing results, particularly in patients with interstitial cystitis. This experience was expressed in a paper read at a regional urological society and eventually led to a book on nutrition called *Food Heal: Why Certain Foods Help YOU Feel Your Best,* which contrasts the matter science diet approach with the energy science nutritional approach, helping the reader understand the differences between the two healing traditions.

I have come to realize that how we view the body can have a profound impact on healing it. This book series is to help show you how applying the knowledge in *Foods Heal* along with the multitude of energy science healing techniques can can help deal with the chronic diseases such as IC and its sister diseases of chronic prostatitis, irritable bowel syndrome (IBS), gastroesophageal reflux disease (GERD), and fibromyalgia. This is my offering to you, dear reader.

In the end, the reason for this book is quite simple. It is to explain and contrast the matter and energy science approaches to disease, which are distinctly different. Hence the energy science approach offers the IC patient a real alternative, not just another matter science therapy.

For those who are interested in a different approach, this can be healing by getting out of the same worn-out rut. "If you keep on doing what you're doing, then you'll keep on getting what you're getting."

Introduction

The real act of discovery consists not in finding new lands but in seeing with fresh eyes.

—Marcel Proust

Chronic disease is a formidable challenge to anyone's life, especially when it involves ongoing, unrelenting pain. No one wants that for anyone. To be condemned to such an existence without hope is one of the most unfortunate things to happen in a person's lifetime.

So this is a book of hope and about how to relieve that pain and give you back the freedom to dream and ecstatic life that you want. It's about reassurance that IC can be healed with a different healing approach so that you can be relieved of your fears and anxiety about this chronic disease. It's about giving you the confidence that this is not a hopeless condition and nothing can be done.

This gives you a basic understanding of the clinical application of the energy science of Ayurveda and helps you understand how it can heal with radical transformative work, IC and its chronic sister diseases such as, GERD, IBS, fibromyalgia, and chronic prostatitis. In this context then IC becomes not only treatable but curable. It looks at these diseases with a different set of glasses than you are currently using.

The use of the energy science approach to disease has a long tradition that has stood the test of time to bring you what you need if you are to become empowered to heal yourself. It offers a systematic scientific approach to chronic disease since it understands the origin of disease.

This book will give you the tools to aid you in healing yourself. But there's one more thing that this book gives you. It's the secret to amazing health. You see, it's not about healing your chronic disease but what happens after you've done that.

The Biologic Simultaneity of Matter and Energy

Einstein's famous equation changed the way you manage your world. The world of physics with $E=mc^2$ and quantum theory was a paradigm shift in thinking that enabled us to put people on the moon and advance computer technology, among many other scientific achievements. But our biological model is still stuck in seeing the body as purely a matter or molecular field.

The equation posits that energy and matter are completely interchangeable at a constant. It states that the biological world is both matter and energy and that your body is simultaneously a matter and an energy field.

So your body is both particle and wave. As a particle, it expresses itself as a molecule. But when you put on your energy field glasses, you see your body as a wave. Indeed, when IC first expresses itself, its symptoms come and go over time as waves, which are called flares.

Currently, the matter science discipline of healing dominates. It is a molecular way of dealing with disease. The energy science medical discipline helps you see disease and its management in a new way. In so doing, you gain a way of healing chronic disease.

Ayurveda: Traditional Indian Medicine

Ayurveda is a five-thousand-year-old medical tradition that comes from the yoga tradition and is a science of healing like the traditional Chinese medicine (TCM) discipline from which is derived the practice of acupuncture. These traditions saw the body as an energy field and used words you may recognize, such as *prana, chi, qi, ru,* and *ruha,* to denote the energy field with which the discipline was working.

Throughout this book series, the term *energy science* is used in contrast to the contemporary matter or molecular science of healing. It is used for two reasons. The first is to note that Ayurveda, like TCM, is a valid medical science. But these traditions do their science differently from the present matter science tradition. Because it's different does not lessen the science's approach, and it's important to know the differences between the two disciplines.

Both are deep philosophical systems, but they articulate their principles of healing and teachings in a cultural way. To try to combine them for personal use is, I believe, a mistake. Choose one system and learn it well. Better to dig one twenty-foot hole than two ten-foot holes.

Secondly, you learn by contrast, and contrasting the matter and energy science approaches allows you to understand more of each one.

It's important to note that I'm using energy science as a very specific term that is not "new age" or "high tech." Although there is a lot of buzz about "energy work," this is not what I mean about the energy science traditions. Although these recent styles of energy work have their application and value, they may not come from deep philosophical foundations as the giants of energy science do.

The intent of this work is to be true to the classic Ayurvedic tradition and its teachings and to show how it has deep relevance for our matter science healing tradition of today.

Natural Healing: Change the Model and Change the Healing of the IC Syndrome

The past two decades have seen a public frustrated with the current matter science approach, as people intuitively believe that health is more than a visit to the doctor. You are no longer willing to give up your responsibility for your health. But how do you take control?

Acceptance of alternative or complementary therapies for managing chronic disease has occurred because matter science has been helpful only to some degree. But amidst this acceptance is confusion. Which alternative therapy is best and for what specific condition? Which herb should I take and for how long?

I believe you as a health consumer want your responsibility back, but the matter science discipline has been telling you that if you want healing, you need to come to one its practitioners. Even though you are exploring health food stores and online health products, you may often have little understanding of what to buy and how to use your purchases.

One of the explicit purposes of this book series is to give you basic, fundamental energy science tools, such as nutritional and lifestyle behavioral work, that will help you heal your disease and promote future health. This kind of information can be empowering. But it comes from understanding the differences between the matter and energy science models.

These sciences do their healing in different ways. In the matter science model, molecules or bacteria cause disease, and treatment involves molecular forms such as pharmaceuticals or surgery. The technological aspects of the matter science approach are indeed impressive.

But where the molecular science approach dashes our hopes for relief of our suffering is in the realm of chronic diseases, such as the IC bladder syndrome. The origins of disease will never be known from a molecular level. The reason for this is quite simple. Disease begins in the energy field and percolates up to the matter field to become expressed as diagnosable.

The energy science model sees disease as an imbalance of qualities that originates most commonly from the GI tract. Hence real healing of chronic disease requires that you eradicate the reason why the disease began in the first place. This requires a different way of healing, so this book becomes one of hope for relieving some of the suffering IC bladder syndrome patients have.

Thinking Outside the Box of Healing

Currently, the alternative medical movement is doing matter science medicine alternatively, and complementary medicine complements the discipline's molecular approach. But there is no structured, systematic way of viewing disease in a different way. So we just keep using the same old disease model in alternative ways.

But when you practice in the energy science medical discipline, you participate in a biological paradigm shift. You step out of the biological Newtonian physics of the past and embark on a journey into the biological energy realm, where real healing can occur. You merge your energy field into the greater energy field you call Nature.

"Perhaps the greatest barrier to a paradigm shift, in some cases, is the reality of paradigm paralysis: the inability or refusal to see beyond the current models of thinking."

—Wikipedia

But you may ask, "Why do I need a model? Is it not enough to know that chamomile tea is effective for relief of an IC flare or that aloe vera gel can be helpful in reducing the number and intensity of IC flares?" Being a pragmatist about healing certainly does the trick at times, but I would submit that this limits the options open for actually healing chronic disease and IC specifically.

When the current matter science dabbles in the energy world of healing, it leads to 1) disorganized, hit-and-miss therapeutic options, 2) a less than satisfactory platform for interpreting results, 3) a lack of understanding of what happened for the better or worse, and 4) lack of trust to be dedicated to long-term healing, which is required in chronic disease. For example, the use of chamomile tea is useful in IC. In the matter science world, that's great, but it's not understood what happened.

Without understanding the basis of a model's approach to healing, there is a lack of knowing why certain foods cause flares for some and not for others. Without a model, there is confusion about why certain foods should not be combined with others. In the end, without an understanding of the energy model, there can be lack of trust and incomplete use of all the potential energy science healing modalities, of which there are many.

This lack of trust becomes a problem when trying to solve chronic disease. Chronic diseases have had a long time to develop, and many times the best that any healer can offer is palliation or to make the patient comfortable. And the energy science of Ayurveda clearly has many tools that can be used to help in this regard. But without trust there will be a natural human tendency to give up on therapies and not continue.

Lack of perseverance is one of the most difficult challenges confronting those with chronic disease. A model that supports continued work in the direction of improved health, even though it's palliative, gives **subtle** cues to the sufferer that things are improving, that life is slowly getting better, and that there will be an end to the disease.

There is the possibility for curing channel diseases such as IC, IBS, and GERD, but even in these situations, radical transformation is necessary for healing to take place.

This is not a simple process, but it's clearly not impossible. It is in this vein that one can say that IC is curable, not just treatable, but you have to understand the context.

Lastly as seen with matter science therapies the use of multiple therapies in the energy science is important. In the matter science oral medications for various targeted benefits, bladder instillations, and hydrodistention procedures are offered for control of symptoms.

The energy science uses the concept of multiple therapies as well but a key distinguishing feature is that a shift in nutrition and metabolic lifestyle behavior patterns is fundamental to healing without which targeted herbal therapies whether orally or through bladder instillations are significantly less effective. Anyone interested in dealing with chronic disease must be willing to take on these challenges.

Lifestyle Choices and Shape-Shifting Your DNA

Mind is no longer neatly tucked away in the brain. It has escaped, and the energy science tells us that the gross expression of mind is the DNA in every cell of the mindbody. And you know that the mind can be flexible, plastic, and malleable, and DNA is that as well. That is why the **hot, sharp/penetrating** qualities of chili peppers can make your mind judgmental, critical, and irritable. On the other hand the **gross, heavy, dull,** and **cold** qualities of cheese or ice cream cause the mind to become **heavy, dull**, depressed, and/or sleepy. And this is all mediated through food's effect on your DNA through the food's qualities.

According to the energy science model, if you make balancing choices, you will correct imbalances and move toward greater states of health. For example, if you make balancing choices around nutrition, your DNA hears that, shape-shifts, and supports the correction of the imbalance in inner space. It does this through qualities in the mindbody. If you take aloe vera gel for the **cold** quality for your IC flares due to **hot** inflammation, your DNA will literally cool off its expression.

This is a valid way of seeing mind and its relationship to disease that helps you understand why any stimulus, whether food, pharmaceutical, herb, environmental influences, or action, can produce a healing or disruptive change to the mindbody. And it's mediated through the mind or DNA. This understanding also shows you how you got the IC bladder syndrome in the first place.

Making unbalancing choices that produce inflammation causes DNA to express the IC bladder syndrome—or, for that matter, any disease—throughout the entire mindbody. So in the end, the syndrome is a systemic disease crafted in your DNA, and any choice that bestows more physiologic balance is a step toward healing, causing a shift in your DNA. In other words, you are in charge of your destiny, and that includes IC.

Are Diseases Woven Together?

The matter science model deals with labels to fit symptoms to the label. For example, if there are symptoms of urgency with pain, burning on urination, urinary frequency, and a negative urine culture, the most likely diagnosis is IC. A label has been given.

But currently the matter science probings are finding that these disease labels seem to be associated. For example, IBS is associated with IC seventy-nine percent of the time, GERD fifty percent, and that chronic prostatitis is equal to its frequency in women(are they the same disease?).

From an energy view, disease is the play of the imbalances of the energy patterns of Vata, Pitta, and Kapha (VPK) in the body, so all diseases become interconnected. Why is this valuable? Since chronic prostatitis, GERD, IBS, and fibromyalgia are also caused by the same energy patterns of VPK, there is an interconnectivity to these disease processes, which enables the energy science to treat all imbalances—not just IC—with the focus of therapy not on the disease label but on the imbalance.

Many have intuited that IC bladder syndrome is a systemic disease, but there is no good explanation from the current matter science approach. In the energy science medical model, all disease arises from the gastrointestinal tract due to imbalances of qualities from foods consumed. This helps us understand that indeed IC is a systemic disease with imbalances occurring in different areas of the body, such as in the case of fibromyalgia.

Energy Science Tools

As you may know, nutrition is the foundation of management for IC and, for that matter, any chronic disease. But diet, which is a matter science term, is different from nutrition. Diet is a molecular (vitamins, fatty acids) and quantitative (calories) evaluation of food eaten.

The energy science approach is much more than a diet approach. It takes into consideration not only the foods ingested from a qualitative aspect, but also many other areas in the greater realm of nutrition—for example, when to take the biggest meal of the day, what foods are incompatible with each other, what is a normal bowel pattern, why digestive strength is important in overall health, what are healthy metabolic lifestyle choices, and how to cultivate a strong digestive system.

But the energy science approach to nutrition only scratches the surface as to other modalities of treatment for IC and other chronic diseases—for example, the use of breathing techniques and yoga poses to improve the strength of digestion, the use of spices in helping with digestion, the use of herbs to help bring balance, the use of oils such as castor oil packs, the use of herbs vaginally for painful intercourse, and the use of specific foods that enhance balance and clear the body of stagnant energy.

Theory Versus Work: The Bottom Line

If you have IC or its sister chronic diseases, the theoretical basis discussed in this book for using the energy science approach may not be appealing. "Just stop these flares!" may be the order of the day. In this situation, go to the appendix of the book and begin right now to take care of your flares.

But I would suggest that as you develop more control of your IC symptoms, exploring other energy science tools can expand your results. So let's get started!

All of the quotes in the book are from patients with IC who wanted to share their story in some way.

Chapter 1

A Story of Interstitial Cystitis and Chronic Disease

"Interstitial cystitis takes a toll on my soul."

Interstitial cystitis (IC) is a chronic noninfectious inflammatory disease of the pelvis and urinary bladder with unknown cause, according to the prevailing matter or molecular science model. It can also adversely affect other adjacent organs, causing symptoms in the vagina, prostate, and lower rectum. The reported number of four million underestimates its true incidence.

From an energy science view, it is not possible to estimate the true incidence because from 50 to 70 percent of sufferers resolve spontaneously with some work. Of these patients, some continue to have symptoms but limp along controlled by occasional hydrodistention or other forms of matter science therapies. The remaining 30 to 40 percent of patients unfortunately develop chronic flare patterns of various severity.

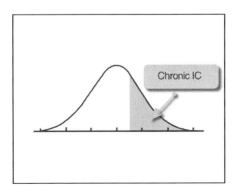

Those who specialize in gynecology estimate that it affects about 16 to 18 percent of all reproductive-age women in America. That means that about one out of every six women between ages fourteen and fifty have some degree of IC, "painful bladder syndrome (PBS)," or chronic pelvic pain syndrome (CPPS).

From an energy science view, it is not possible to estimate the true incidence because in actuality the disease presents as a spectrum ranging from those who have a brief series of flares that resolve spontaneously to those who develop chronic debilitating symptoms at various severity levels.

Men labeled with the diagnosis of chronic prostatitis in the past may have responded to IC-type treatment. Incidence figures do not include children, who are also affected by symptoms. Unexplained changes in childhood voiding patterns, particularly those predisposed by their makeup with negative workups, are invariably IC.

IC is also associated with diseases such as GERD, IBS, and fibromyalgia. But as you will see, there is a definite energetic relationship among these diseases. Hence low-grade urinary symptoms with patients who have these problems are usually indicative of IC. In short, from all of the above the IC bladder syndrome is a common health problemSometimes the imbalance leading to the IC bladder syndrome can be cleared by simple measures. Some estimate returns to a state of balance and spontaneous resolution occurrences to be as high as 50 percent. Most important, the remaining group of women and men go on to chronic debilitating IC symptoms.

As would seem obvious, the longer the imbalance continues over the years and decades, the greater the likelihood that more diligent measures need to be undertaken for a longer period in order for physiologic balance to be restored.

Chronic Disease

As opposed to *acute,* which refers to an immediate issue such as acute appendicitis, acute cholecystitis, or an acute bacterial bladder infection, the term *chronic disease* implies a lingering ailment that has no specific solution and is often said to be treatable but not curable. At times, the acute flare of IC is interpreted as an acute bacterial infection, but in light of the recurrent nature of the "infections," it is a chronic illness. Hence chronic diseases have intermittent acute exacerbations, such as the flare in IC or the painful acceleration of joint symptoms in rheumatoid arthritis.

By making this separation of acute and chronic, the matter science medical model establishes that there are disease states that can be healed (acute) and those that cannot be healed (chronic). The energy science medical model makes no distinction. **This is basically due to the understanding of the origin of disease.** The molecular model still seeks the origin, whereas from the energy model side the origins are clear—an imbalance is affecting the physiology.

From an energy science view, all diseases are potentially curable, but significant efforts on the part of the affected are required. In the case of IC, healing is possible, as it is not a tissue layer but a urinary channel problem.

But as the saying goes, there's no free lunch. Real healing requires time and directed effort. **This is a marked departure from our current worldview of chronic disease.**

If you have a lingering disease, the response is all too often shades of "too bad, "bit of bad luck", "too bad for you", and "I'll pray for you." As you will see, the impact that chronic disease such as IC has on those who are suffering is dramatic and significant. Compassion due to this suffering leads healers to look for means to help.

How Do I Know I Have IC?

The symptoms of IC are painful urgency for needing to urinate, frequency of urination (every fifteen to twenty-five minutes) and typically burning on urination (dysuria), or lower abdominal pain that occurs on a periodic basis. These symptoms together cause you and your doctor to think you have a urinary tract infection (UTI), but in the case of IC, the urine culture is negative. What marks the chronic course of IC is that there are repetitive symptom episodes, called flares, lasting typically two to three weeks, sometimes shorter or longer. It is typical that between two and seven years lapse before the diagnosis of IC is made.

Mary's story is typical of the matter science medical evaluation for what turns out to be IC. It is not meant to be a criticism of this model of healing but to illustrate the current lack of understanding of the chronic disease process.

Mary is a thirty-eight-year-old married redheaded woman with no specific ethnicity who develops frequency, urgency, and burning involving urination. She has two teenage children. The symptom complex becomes bothersome without relief from suggested home remedies that include drinking lots of fluids and cranberry juice. This seems to help some but does not resolve her problems of voiding frequency and pain.

The experience brings back her childhood memories of UTIs and frequent urination. Although never urologically evaluated, she felt growing up that her bladder was a weak area of her body. After she began menstruating at age thirteen, her bladder symptoms seemed to become less of a problem.

She goes to her family physician, who diagnoses a UTI by voided urine. She is given antibiotics for three days, and this seems to relieve her symptoms but not entirely. Because of that, she continues to use the cranberry juice and pushes fluids. After about another week, she gradually resolves her symptom complex.

Mary once again develops the recurrence of the same symptom complex that she had two years before (time intervals can vary significantly). She begins the methods she used in the past but again has no complete relief. Her physician bases the diagnosis of UTI once again on a urinalysis (urine examination under a microscope) and prescribes antibiotics once more.

Now fast-forward one year. Mary has now had two more episodic symptom complexes after the one last year. She is growing weary of the repetitive nature of the problem and asks her physician, **"What's wrong with my bladder that it continues to get infected?"** She is given information about voiding after intercourse and provided antibiotics for a full two weeks with talk about the possibility of a suppressive course of antibiotics in the future.

The Trip to the Gynecologist

The family practitioner discusses the situation with Mary, and they agree that a female (gynecological) evaluation should be done to be sure she does not have endometriosis or some other genital problem. She sees the gynecologist and there seems to be tenderness over the uterine area, but she has just finished a course of antibiotics.

Routine studies such as PAP smears, cultures, and hormonal levels are performed. The reports come back as normal. A pelvic ultrasound is done for more exacting information about her uterine cavity and size. Again this reveals nothing abnormal, but the pelvic exam still shows some tenderness.

Another course of antibiotics has no effect on the specific tenderness, so an endometrial biopsy is done. This is negative. Later the gynecologist performs a laparoscopy and burns points on the internal lining of the abdomen, thinking that these are signs of endometriosis. After recovery from the anesthesia and the exam, Mary thinks she feels better, and she is labeled with the diagnosis of endometriosis. She is given a trial of a drug to suppress the endometrium but over time has no change in her episodic symptoms.

Three months later Mary begins experiencing the same symptoms that she had before she saw the gynecologist, and now it becomes clear that her bladder is the problem, not endometriosis. Thousands of dollars later, she is no closer to what's going on than when she started. She feels mounting frustration and anger.

Mary becomes disenchanted with the advice thus far and seeks another physician's opinion with her next recurrence of symptoms. She relates that she has had five UTIs documented by urinalyses and treated with antibiotics. This time a urine culture shows an organism that is sensitive to the antibiotics chosen. It seems to clear her symptoms, and she is treated with a full two weeks of antibiotics. Now she is placed on a suppressive antibiotic dosing for a month, taking one pill a day.

In review: Mary began having UTIs a little over three years ago, and despite many short-term courses of antibiotics, she continued to have these recurrent symptom complexes of "UTI." There has not been culture documentation of infection until recent. Her symptom complexes seem to be getting more frequent (less time between flares), and the symptoms take longer to resolve. The repeated and untimely nature of these flares interpreted as bacterial UTIs are wearing on her emotionally. After the extensive negative gynecological evaluation, she has become frustrated and angry that there seems to be no resolution to what she is now seeing as a chronic problem.

A Visit to the Urologist

In this progressive medical drama, on the next symptom complex, her physician does a urine culture, which shows no bacterial growth. She is given antibiotics, but due to the negative urine culture, an appointment is made with a urologist. The course of antibiotics seems to help with the clearance of symptoms again.

Her urology appointment involves a detailed history of her past "infections" as well as other past medical history. She has a thorough physical exam with a urine culture done on a catheterized specimen (small tube is placed into the bladder to collect a urine specimen). The passage of the catheter by the nurse is painful.

She is instructed to come back when she has symptoms and given a prescription for Elmiron. A telephone call from the office reports no evidence of infection. In the interim she undergoes a CT scan of the kidneys and bladder, with no significant findings.

Mary returns for the results of the testing one month after her initial visit and to report on how the Elmiron worked. She has no symptoms, but she is not sure what to expect.

One week later Mary begins to have UTI symptoms. A catheterized specimen is obtained, causing a lot of pain, and she is given antibiotics. The culture returns with no bacterial growth, indicating she has no infectious process causing her symptom complex.

Now in review: Mary has had recurrent symptom complexes of an apparent "UTI" for 3½ years with a negative gynecological evaluation. She now has a history of negative urine cultures with symptoms supporting the diagnosis of IC with negative urine cultures and a normal x-ray exam of the urinary tract. Mary has the diagnosis of IC by exclusion. One last exam would further establish the IC diagnosis.

Treatable but Not Curable

Mary returns after she is more comfortable with antibiotics and the Elmiron, although her symptoms now do not seem to completely clear as they had in the past. The urologist gives her two options. She can have a potassium chloride stimulation test that may be equivocal or have an evaluation of the bladder lining with a flexible endoscope. Due to microscopic blood in the urine seen in the past, he suggests a cystoscopy.

She elects to have the cystoscopy (look into the bladder), which is the most painful thing she has had to endure thus far in this bladder journey. Glomerulations are seen with pseudomembranous formation on the trigone but no Hunner's ulcer(s). A prescription of pain medication is given, and it takes her three days to recover from the experience. The value is that the exam does not disclose any abnormality.

Mary receives an antidepressant from her sympathetic urologist, who proceeds to tell her about IC and relates that **the condition "is treatable but not curable."** Mary has a heavy portending feeling in her stomach as she hears these words. She feels as if she has just been given a lifelong sentence without parole.

"Unfortunately, there is little that medical science can provide for you but empathy, compassion, and pharmaceutical support," her urologist relates.

"The problem, Mary, is that we don't know what causes this disease," the urologist explains. "As yet there's no molecular marker to track, although research suggests that we may be close. APF (antiproliferative factor) and AMP (antimicrobial peptides) are potential molecules involved in the disease."

"What does a marker or molecule mean for me?" Mary asked. "Since I have IC, what does a molecule mean?"

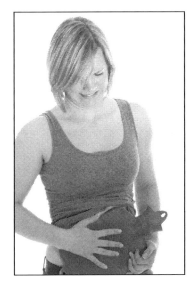

"Well, if we have a marker specific to IC, that may become a molecular portal or window to explain the origin of the disease itself. That's the idea, anyway.

"But we have a lot of various drugs that can help you make the symptoms bearable so you can live a somewhat normal life."

Somewhat normal life? Mary thought. *What does that mean?*

Now in review: After an early childhood experience of urinary voiding issues cleared with menstruation, Mary at age forty-two has now had intermittent symptoms complexes of IC for four years with a negative gynecological exam and now a urological evaluation with endoscopy that is consistent with IC. Glomerulations and pseudomembranous formation of the trigone are the observations without Hunner's ulcers, which are typically infrequent. "Treatable but not curable" is the message, and she begins pharmaceutical trials to see what works best for her.

Mary's Plight

With this information, Mary is glad she has the antidepressant and goes home crying and feeling sad and lonely. Many thoughts race through her mind. At least she does not have cancer. Or perhaps that would be better. Then at least she would have a "disease label" to treat.

She begins doing Internet IC research, looking for threads she may find to help her cope with this condition. She finds a lot on diet and learns that certain "trigger foods" may be the answer to reducing these flares that were once called "UTIs." But she also finds confusing information that does not give her much understanding about the condition.

Mary does find two important support systems that have been created for people with IC. The Interstitial Cystitis Association (ICA: http://www.ichelp.org/page.aspx?pid=585) and the Interstitial Cystitis Network (ICN: http://www.ic-network.com/support/#supportgroups) provide not only group support in local communities but also have discussion threads on various topics at their websites. Mary finds a support group locally that provides her educational material and answers her questions. But more than this, Mary has a group of understanding and compassionate friends who know what she is going through.

Matter Science Therapies

Mary's symptoms become worse as the years progress. At times she is not able to get out of bed due to the pain during flares. She becomes sick of being sick, and she feels robbed of something that normal people take for granted. And she experiences all the emotions a normal person would in such a situation, from anger, frustration, and confusion to hopelessness and alienation.

Early on she is tried on oxybutynin and it has little impact on her frequency and urgency but gives her a dry mouth. Other anticholinergics and anti-inflammatories are tried but nothing clears the symptoms. Mary then hears of people who can't urinate with these drugs and elects to not do any of them as not being able to urinate scares her.

With the information on diet she gathered from the Internet and friends in her support group, Mary begins adjusting her approach to food and sees that there are definite "triggers" that lead to flares. But there seems to be disconnects because some foods that are not labeled as triggers act as such for her. This diet work seems to make a big difference for her.

Mary begins a series of six weekly DMSO instillations to the bladder, but after going through the second instillation, she cannot endure any more treatments. The intense pain lays her up for two days after each treatment. "The treatment is worse than the cure," she muses. She begs off on any further local therapies.

As the months go by, Mary finds that the Elmiron seems to be effective in reducing the intensity of the flare. She is less clear about the other drugs but will try anything to help with the pain but the hair loss is sad and she wonders about stopping the Elmiron.

At the suggestion of her urologist, Mary begins a physical therapy program to "learn about the pelvic floor" and how this might play a role in her symptom complex. After eight weeks, she has more knowledge about the perineal area but is unconvinced that this information will reduce her flares. Another avenue explored.

Mary also learns from her IC support group about an InterStim implant. She hears mixed reviews. Some felt no better but others had remarkable results. She elects to hold off on the technique, which would require an additional operative procedure.

After exploring many avenues, a harsh reality that there is nothing available sets in for Mary. With each new disappointment comes a sense of hopelessness and despair about clearance of this condition. She develops an overwhelming frustration and disillusioned because all the therapies work for a while then stop working, or don't work at all. Sometimes she feels like an experiment.

Mary also explores injections of Botox into the bladder muscle wall to see if this can help her symptoms. Although she seemed to have some relief early on after a several injection sessions the effect wore off and so she stopped.

Relationships

Mary's IC medical story is only one aspect of the impact this chronic disease has on Mary's life. To fully understand its effect, it is helpful to know what happens to Mary's social life due to this chronic disease. As you may recall, Mary has a teenage boy and girl. Both are very active in school functions and sports.

As Mary's IC flares become more involved, she has less involvement with her children. **The urgency of trying to make it to a bathroom would lead to unbearable bladder pain.** From a matter science medical understanding, the disease process of IC involves the bladder wall and its nerve endings.

Pain in the lower pelvic area over the bladder region occurs when the bladder becomes stretched to any small degree. So to keep the pain to a tolerable level, Mary had to seek out bathrooms or portable toilets at functions such as soccer games. The daily interference of normal activities with her kids was disheartening to Mary, but she had no choice but to begin to curtail her activities around her children's functions.

The emotional pain of not being able to grow with her children was one thing, but it was more than that. Mary began having a sense of guilt that she should be doing something about her IC, but she had no idea what that might be. Intuitively she had a sense that there were things that could be done to alleviate the problem, which fed on her guilt.

Mary's relationships with her immediate family became a challenge as they had never heard of IC and could not understand why she was so "picky" about her food choices during gatherings. She appeared outwardly healthy, so what was the problem? Again Mary wished that she had a serious illness such as cancer so at least there would be empathy about her disease.

She not only lost out on her children's activities, but her social friendships with her girlfriends also began to slowly erode. The urgency pain interfered with her day-to-day schedule on a regular basis. Mary found her worst time was being "trapped in a car." She would be with a friend and have to ask her to pull over at various restrooms along the way because of the pain.

As a result, she finds herself isolated and lonely. **Mary finds that her best friends are her IC support group because at least they understand the pain that she is going through.** At times she becomes very depressed, but her support group becomes "her group of strength."

With continued painful flares, Mary finds that she cannot attend to her job as a receptionist at a local company. Due to the absenteeism, she is finally let go, which is probably the most compassionate thing that her employer could do. But for Mary it becomes just another loss, leading to more isolation.

Sex and Intimacy

Sexual relationships with Mary's husband of twenty years are lost. Although appreciating Mary's affection and attempts, Jake becomes uncomfortable in causing her pain. Her fear of pain begins to mix with the fear of losing her relationship. But now just the thought of intercourse during foreplay will cause her to break into a **cold** sweat due to her anxiety.

The lower abdominal pain that radiated into her thighs gradually became unbearable. And the after effects of intercourse with flare like symptoms and severe urgency led her to avoid intimacy at all. No one likes to labeled as **cold** or aloof but Mary really had no choice.

Mary and Jake had always enjoyed a healthy sex life, and this loss was very difficult for both of them. She was so grateful for his understanding and sticking it out with her. Trying different positions, extended foreplay, and induced orgasms in creative ways became their solution. It brought for her new meaning to the vows of "in sickness and in health," since she had heard of other women whose husbands had divorced over this disease.

Mary had someone in her support group with a condition called vulvodynia, which causes such intense vaginal pain that it is virtually impossible for women to have intercourse. The bladder lies on the front part of the vagina, so it is not surprising that many cases of vulvodynia are related to IC.

For Mary, there was a feeling of worthlessness, a sense that she had become in some way "damaged goods." She felt a loss of womanhood, similar to the loss felt by men with impotence. She was an attractive woman but could not perform.

She had heard of women who feared sex because of the possibility of getting pregnant. Would they be able to take their meds during pregnancy? Would they be able to manage the pregnancy? Would they be able to care for their child after birth?

IC and Chronic Disease Anxiety

Chronic illness has many faces, but the one that is most troubling is that it's always there. But not all chronic illnesses are created equally with respect to pain. Chronic illness is one thing, but chronic illness with unrelenting pain is tormenting.

When we are not feeling well, there is most often for all of us a fear of whether things will get better—the fear of uncertainty. This particularly becomes the case with chronic disease associated with unrelenting pain. Will I ever be pain free again?

A disease's unknown factors bring fear to any of us. Will this pain ever go away? Will my symptoms get worse? Will there be permanent damage as a result of this disease? How long will it take for this pain to go away? Is my body falling apart? Are other organs being damaged? Will I have to live the rest of my life with this condition?

Chronic fatigue occurs with chronic disease because the energy expended in dealing with daily pain leads to exhaustion. The use of power naps become the norm in order for the body to "catch up." Often it's not choice, the body simply demands that rest is required.

And you may have to pass up the events that you look forward to due to the unpredictable whims of the chronic problem. Missing your daughter's wedding due to a flare becomes a real anxiety now, not something born in the imagination. Or the cancellation of long-awaited trip due to IC leads you to not make any plans at all. Why bother?

The anxiety that the pain of IC will never go away is daunting. And what happens if the painful symptoms get worse? Is there progressive damage being done to my bladder? Where can I turn for help? Yes, there are narcotics and pharmaceuticals such as antidepressants, but they do not take the pain away.

The Sister Diseases

As Mary moved along with disease progression, she found that bowel problems began showing up. She had experienced symptoms of gastroesophageal reflux disease (GERD) even before the first "UTI," but with baking soda or over-the-counter Tums or Rolaids, the heartburn would resolve quickly.

But as the years progressed after the IC diagnosis, she would experience intermittent diarrhea and constipation. The diarrhea was severe at first and seemed to be related to her flares. But as the years passed, constipation became the norm.

She heard of "leaky gut syndrome" as part of the process of the bowel side of IC, and it seemed like a different problem (as you will see in later chapters, there is a defined correlation of bowel problems and IC; intolerances to foods containing gluten and lactose also appear to be unrelated but from an energy view completely understandable).

Although Mary had no specific joint pains, she did have friends who had been given the label of fibromyalgia. With further research, she found an association between IC and this painful muscle and joint condition of unknown cause.

And now Mary learns that men with "chronic prostatitis" may have IC. It would make sense that men would also be affected. Why would IC be sexist? But of course if the prostate is there, why not blame that organ for the symptoms? It's like vulvodynia. If it's there, why not blame the vagina for the pain? It seemed to Mary that a "blame game" was being used since no one knew.

The 5 IC Myths

1. IC is a condition that is limited to the pelvis and bladder.

As discussed previously, there are sister diseases of IC that indicate systemic changes are occurring, leading to the localization of changes in the pelvis and specifically the bladder. Surrounding organs may also be drawn into this energetic process, such as the lower rectum, prostate, and vagina. But the association of IBS, GERD, and fibromyalgia indicate that IC is part of a systemic process or syndrome.

2. Presence of bacteria eliminates the diagnosis of IC.

It is clear that a nonspecific nonbacterial inflammatory change can lead to a bacterial infection because the bladder lining's immune status is compromised. This concept is put forth in the accompanying diagram. It shows that inflammation alone can produce bladder symptoms without infection.

But it also demonstrates how inflammation can be the breeding ground for potential infections. With the localization of the involved energy patterns, the bladder mucosa becomes "sick" and the normal bladder defense mechanisms (GAG layer being one of them) are not optimally functioning, leading to the increased probability of a bacteriologically determined "UTI."

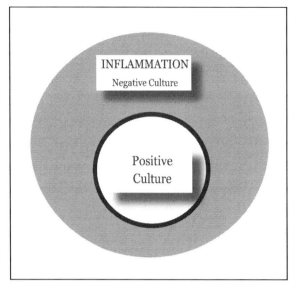

So all patients with IC can get occasional secondary infections, leading to the confusion that UTIs exist and then they do not. Both clinical situations are associated with similar albeit not the same symptoms when carefully observed.

3. Hydrodistention is an important treatment in IC.

Distending a normal organ can cause it to bleed. But distending the inflamed IC bladder can make it bleed significantly, with hemorrhages noted throughout the bladder lining. There is relief with hydrodistention, but for benefit it will have to be repeated in order to forestall repeated symptom complexes.

The energy science understanding of hydrodistention is the temporary paralysis of the bladder muscle, which leads to reduction in frequency, urgency, and even pain. This has no long-term therapeutic value except that it leaves the patient open to bladder wall fibrosis. In a recent policy paper, the American Urological Association (AUA) did not advocate hydrodistention as a therapy for IC.

4. Cystoscopy (exam of the bladder) typically shows abnormal findings.

The diagnostic finding of Hunner's ulcers is an unusual finding, usually 7 percent and primarily in patients who have had IC for many years. This suggests that the presence of ulcers implies longstanding disease. Its absence does not rule out IC. The ulcer should be biopsied to rule out the more serious carcinoma in situ. (http://1.usa.gov/Ys40K8)

If not done under anesthesia, pain during the exam—particularly in the urethra—is a subjective finding but highly suggestive of IC. I believe that pseudomembranous formation of the trigone, although common, is an inflammatory finding in anyone and should be added into the diagnostic summary. Glomerulations as in Mary's story display the inflammatory condition of the bladder.

Many people with glomerulations and trigonal changes have low-grade inflammation that may or may not manifest as IC. The inflammation may show up in other areas of the body as in GERD, IBS, and fibromyalgia.

5. There is a no hormonal association with IC and the menstrual state.

Although there are abundant observations of women reporting changes in symptoms around menses, the matter science has no explanation. As you will see in future chapters, Pitta (**hot** quality), the energy of transformation responsible for IC, is heightened during menopause and causes lack of menstrual flow. Estrogen is a Pitta molecule, and its resultant hormonal effects are Pitta dominant. Monthly menstrual flow is a way of eliminating this energy and its **hot** quality from the physiology. This is why it is commonly reported that IC symptoms worsen prior to menses and then dissipate during menses. With menopause, over time this transformative energy and the **hot** quality leading to IC builds up in those already predisposed.

Energy Science Medical Therapies

There is a growing awareness in the IC communities that the current matter or molecular science discipline may not be the solution to IC. And books such as *The Better Bladder Book* by Wendy Cohan, RN, are challenging the status quo of the current medical care as described in Mary's history.

But you cannot take yourself out of the present environment, where the molecular science approach reigns supreme. Doctors have become the high priest technocrats of the scientific method. And what they say goes because they do save lives in acute medical situations.

The matter science, despite its inadequacies dealing with chronic disease, gets our reverence when it pulls a loved one through a medical crisis. I believe as a health consumer you want to feel at least subconsciously secure in what information you are using as advice to help you with your IC. Why should you trust the fact that aloe vera gel or chamomile tea should be effective in dealing with your IC unless you have personal experience?

Is there not science that supports why energy science therapies work? Yes, the molecular science can help us to see that aloe is made up of long-chain polymers of mannose molecules and that mannose is an "essential glucosacharide" that is helpful in GAG layer formation. That's indeed helpful information.

From my vantage point, trained both in the matter and energy science disciplines, you should expect good science from your healing disciplines in order to understand the rationale of therapies proposed, even if they are about chamomile tea or aloe. But if the energy science does its science differently than the molecular science, should it be discounted?

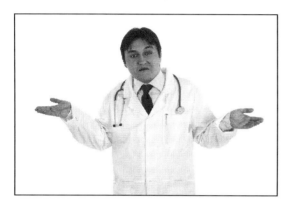

I am a strong advocate of the marriage of these disciplines to improve overall our ability to heal a wider range of health problems. I believe the integration of these two disciplines is the answer to our current medical care stagnation, particularly as it revolves around chronic disease such as IC.

So in a way, the terms *alternative, complementary,* and *holistic* tend to separate rather than support a truly integrated health system that is grounded in seeing the mindbody as a simultaneity of both energy and matter fields. With simultaneity, health problems are not separated, health options are not split, and care is not dependent on something other. Rather, there is a oneness in medical delivery based on which discipline works best in certain situations.

But you should have confidence in this "alternative" energy science medical discipline. And one of the reasons for this book is to give you the scientific understanding of how the energy science arrives at its decision making. To be clear, the matter and energy medical science disciplines do their science in different ways. But just because they do their science differently does not invalidate either approach.

To understand this then brings you confidence that this energy science approach can be helpful in dealing with your chronic disease, and it helps you to see how you should have different expectations from each approach. So let's explore together this approach to healing IC.

Chapter Summary

The actual incidence of IC is unknown, but it is much more than reported numbers. The diagnosis is made by repeated episodes of urinary tract symptoms without evidence of bacteria on urine culture, normal urinary tract radiographic findings, and cystoscopic findings consistent with IC. Although the history usually gives the diagnosis, these studies eliminate other possible pelvic disease.

When it becomes a chronic condition, the bladder syndrome is debilitating in all areas of life due to the unpredictability of flares, poorly controlled pain, and loss of relationships. Loss of sexual intimacy due to pain can potentially damage marriages. And there can be free-floating anxiety related to the chronic disease itself.

Other diseases are associated with IC and are understood when the energy science model is applied. Mythology floats around a diagnosis when the disease is not understood. These myths include beliefs such as secondary bacterial infections exclude the diagnosis of IC or that there is no relationship of menstrual flow and IC. Many different energy science tools can be offered to those with IC that can heal the disease.

So now, let's explore the world of the energy science medical discipline.

Chapter 2

Seeking Balance in All the Right Places

"With cancer you either get better or die. With IC there is no end to the symptoms. Suffering goes on and on. Most chronic diseases don't give symptoms. There is at times tremendous compassion from urologists and doctors, but they can't do anything about it."

The energy body is like a car battery. If you leave the lights on the battery is drained of its stored energy. If you have a chronic disease like IC, the body loses its energy. The result is fatigue, loss of strength and vitality with the constant distraction from symptoms leading to further losses of energy.

Nature's inherent desire is to be in balance. Since you are part of Nature, you know intuitively that balance is important in life, and it speaks to your knowing that balance is something for which you should strive in all areas of your life. From an energy science view, any disease (discomfort, pain, disharmony) is a sign of physiologic energetic imbalance, and the painful flares of IC are expressions of that imbalance.

Imbalance of energetic qualities is the way that the energy science sees disease and how the qualities can bring about systemic disease. Qualities begin to affect not only the urinary tract function, leading to the painful flares of IC, but these same qualities of **hot** and **mobile** begin to cause changes in GI function, leading to the intermittent diarrhea and constipation of irritable bowel syndrome (IBS).

At the stomach level, the **hot** quality in excess leads to hyperacidity syndrome (heartburn) or gastroesophageal reflux disease (GERD). Fibromyalgia occurs when the **hot, dry,** and **rough** qualities lead to pain in the muscle layers of the energy body.

If qualities are in balance, a state of mindbody health is possible. Let's learn more about these qualities in yourself and Nature, for they form the foundation of the energy science medical model.

Nature's Expression as Ten Pairs of Opposing Qualities

In order for you and I to have a dialogue about healing with the energy science of Ayurveda, you will need a vocabulary about this science in order to understand how it is different from what you currently use for health. The first principle is that Nature is made up of ten pairs of contrasting qualities: **heavy/light, dull/sharp, hot/cold, rough/smooth, dry/oily, dense/liquid, hard/soft, subtle/gross, static/mobile,** and **cloudy/clear.**

It is beyond the scope of this book to go into detail about the underlying contemporary science that supports this science of healing. But the prevailing string theory for the unification of all observable energies in the universe states that the universe (Nature) is composed of ten pairs of vibrating strings. The qualities are merely verbal descriptors of each of these strings.

If you and I are part of Nature, which is composed of these fundamental building blocks of energy, you realize that the fresh tomato you eat has the same qualities as you have. If there is a lot of **hot** quality in your biologic energy field, then eating a tomato with the same **hot** quality could give you inflammation and a flare since the excessive **hot** quality produces inflammation. When you pay attention, Nature speaks through these opposing qualities.

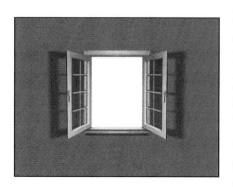

In fact, the qualities are your window of observation of the biological workings of your energy field and Nature herself, because what happens in Nature happens in you. These qualities or vibrational frequencies are footprints of the **subtle** biologic energy field realm. They become signposts as to what is happening in the energy field. And that is the solution to problems: If there is excessive **hot** (inflammation), then finding things to counter with **cold** can be done for healing.

Qualities and the Energy Patterns of Vata, Pitta, and Kapha

Initially, the only way you know that the **hot** quality is excessive is with a flare. **Food is the key factor in producing disease of any kind, including IC, since you consume food on a regular basis**. If foods are consumed unconsciously that produce imbalance, then the result is disease.

You can take all the medicines or herbs in the world, but if you are ignorant about how your own nutrition is causing your imbalance, no medicines or herbs will help you. So you can now see how fundamentally important nutrition is in healing any chronic disease, including IC. The purpose of the energy science nutritional formats that I will share with you is to help guide your food choices.

Although perhaps understood, it is also important to emphasize that simply because you don't feel **hot** that your energy physiology isn't **hot**. And this goes for any of the qualities discussed. At times you may transiently experience a quality but you have to turn up the awareness and attention to the quality to have the experience.

For example, the **slimy/smooth** quality of a spring time cold in the form of mucous is just a cold unless you tune into the energy expression. Or the acid indigestion although experienced as heartburn is just that unless you tune into the experience as a reflection of what's happening in the energy body in terms of the **hot** quality. It is merely changing the perspective of how the interpretation is done.

From these building blocks or qualities are created the energy patterns of Vata (**light, cold, rough, dry, subtle, mobile,** and **clear**), Pitta (**light, sharp, hot, oily, liquid,** and **mobile**), and Kapha (**heavy, dull, cold, smooth, oily, dense, liquid, hard, soft, gross, static,** and **cloudy**). These concepts are explored further in the next chapter.

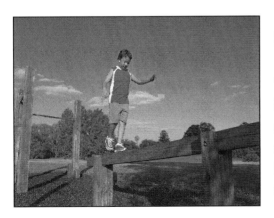

Balance and IC

When it comes to creating health, balance is similar to walking on a gymnastic balance beam. As you walk on the beam by making choices, you right yourself by moving to the left and then to the right in order to remain on the beam. In a similar way, the choices that you make on a moment-to-moment, day-by-day basis biologically put you in balance or out of balance.

If unconsciously you make unbalancing choices over and over again, day after day, month after month, year after year, and decade after decade, eventually you fall off the beam of health and create chronic diseases such as IC, IBS, GERD, and fibromyalgia.

The contemporary molecular or matter science model of healing has no explanation as to why there is an association of IC with these disease labels. And this model will never be able to make that association between them because the link between these seemingly disparate diseases is not a molecular association. The association occurs at the energy level.

Our current molecular or matter field model does not allow you to understand the origins of disease but only to make observations of the results of your chronic unbalancing choices that lead to the painful flares of IC. From a matter field vantage point, you are viewing the tip of the iceberg of chronic unbalancing choices.

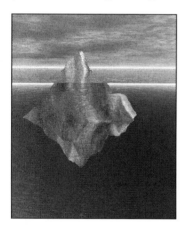

In essence, *balance* means "neutral point," and you know when you are out of balance from the sensations in your body. The energy field of the mindbody wants to be vibrationally balanced. Your digestion is neither too **hot** nor too **cold;** your energetic physiology neither too **mobile** nor too **static;** your energetic mindbody neither too **sharp** nor too **dull;** your energetic metabolism neither too **heavy** nor too **light.**

Mary's Story

*Mary began noticing that when her flares began, she would have a nervous feeling (**mobile**) in her stomach and a feeling of **hot** in the lower pelvis. This would be particularly pronounced about three or four days before her menses began and then would dissipate by the end of menstrual flow. She became aware that there seemed to be a correlation between her diarrhea (**hot**) related to her IBS and her flares. She was now wondering if the drugs she was taking were doing any good.*

Flares and the Bathtub

The unpredictable flares that occur at the most inopportune times are a very distressing aspect of IC. This can be easily understood using the energy science model. Remember that energy expresses itself in Nature as a particle or wave form. As wave forms, whenever vibrational frequency patterns are added in excess to the biological energy physiology, you observe increased oscillations.

Since you are not separate from Nature, the occurrences that you see in Nature mimic what you experience in your own body. It is not a coincidence that the intermittent and unanticipated bladder pains have become known as flares, similar to the intense **hot** solar flares observed from the sun.

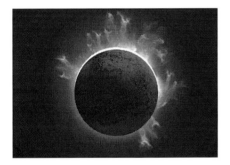

This is characteristic of any disease process with the waxing and waning of symptoms and signs of imbalances occurring in an oscillating pattern. This is precisely the pattern seen in acute and chronic IC.

You can view the energy mindbody at its epicenter, the GI tract, as a bathtub full of water. There is an interface here between your outside energy world, the environment, and you. Specifically, food is at the GI tract interface, where imbalanced and balanced energetic states are created by your choices.

In balance, the energy mindbody is like a placid tub of water without any turbulence. With unbalancing lifestyle choices, primarily as IC inflammatory foods, qualities begin accumulating in the mindbody's GI energy field. You begin to see ripples on the surface of the water as the energetic system begins to accumulate excess qualities. Words such as *accumulation* and *provocation* define a change or disturbance in the status of your GI energy field. Due to the accumulation of excess vibrational frequencies, there is a disturbance in the energy field. An imbalance, disruption, or turmoil is being created in your energy field that I call the bathtub.

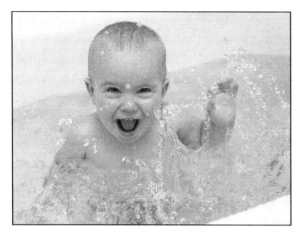

Energetically, prepathological conditions are produced because of the accumulated qualities. You consume foods as qualities that can either produce calmness or bring turmoil to your personal energy field. As months, years, and decades of unbalancing lifestyle choices roll along and the ripples of your bathtub begin to become small waves, you progressively begin to intermittently disseminate this accumulated energy to the urinary tract as in IC.

This begins the symptom complex of IC. Eventually the turbulence becomes so great that the choices culminate into such large waves that they begin to slosh over the sides of the tub, spilling outside the GI tract and localizing on the bathroom floor—or, in this case, your bladder. At this point the energy disruption is severe enough to permanently enter into the urinary channel of the body. **The important observation here is that you are the person making the turbulence.**

Eventually you begin seeing changes to the flooring, and finally, dry rot starts the destructive process of the bathroom floor or bladder. The process begins in unconscious innocent choices, but in the end it destroys the bathroom and the bladder is left in a state of chronic disease. This energetic disruption of your urinary bladder creates the chronic changes and symptoms of IC.

GI Tract Provocation and IC

So from this biological model, you can see how the GI tract is fundamental to the health of the body. This is why IC is associated with IBS and GERD. The unbalanced qualities in the GI tract lead to other chronic GI diseases. By making the correct lifestyle choices around eating, you can create and maintain balance in your physiology by understanding your relationship with the foods that you consume.

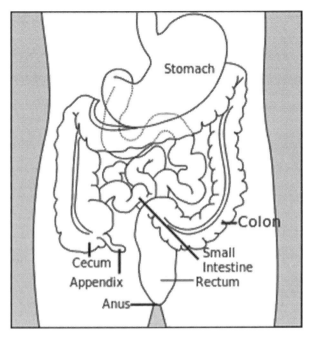

The matter field system lacks understanding as to the importance of the GI tract health. And even if there is some understanding, consensus as to how to achieve that status of health is lacking. **If the GI tract is sick, pharmaceuticals, supplements, and herbs cannot be absorbed effectively if you keep making the same energetic food mistakes over and over again.**

When you truly understand this concept, you have made an evolutionary step forward in your health. If you elect to perpetuate your matter field nutritional mistakes, you will continue your downward spiral in the management of chronic diseases such as IC. There are direct energetic physiologic consequences of food that can promote balance or imbalance.

For example, if you as a PV (Pitta/Vata—next chapter) already have **hot, mobile,** and **dry** qualities and you add more **hot, mobile,** and **dry** qualities in the form of salsa and corn tortilla chips, there will no doubt over the days, months, years, and decades an accumulation and provocation with dissemination of these qualities.

These qualities potentially manifest on the skin as **hot, mobile,** and **dry,** spreading lesions, or internally with **hot, mobile,** and **dry** symptoms of bladder irritation, experienced as burning on urination (**hot**) and urinary frequency (**mobile**) unassociated with bacterial infection. If antibiotics are used, they may be effective in reducing the inflammatory symptoms, since antibiotics are anti-inflammatory in nature.

The problem for you is that there is such variability in the time lag between ingestion and manifestation of imbalance that you have a hard time believing that, when you have an energy makeup of PV, routinely eating corn, tomato, or cranberry has anything to do with your bladder symptoms.

The important energetic effect of food is that the qualities ingested have physiologic consequences that linger for thirty-five days. The heartburn may dissipate twenty-four hours later after a provoked PV has ingested **hot** and **mobile** salsa with corn chips, but energetically the qualities of the provocation linger through the tissues for much longer.

Progression of the IC Imbalance

From an allopathic or matter science medical view, when a disease is diagnosed in effect a label is placed on the tip of the iceberg. But there is so much more energetically to the disease below the surface.

This implies that our energy fields are being provoked from very early in our lives. As you grow in years, potentially more qualities accumulate in your energy body but then are shed. The buildup of an imbalanced quality may require years and years of unbalancing choices that are small but incremental and cumulative.

Mary's Story
In retrospect even though Mary was "asymptomatic" between her intial UTI's she now recalls that her intermittent diarrhea, skin rashes, and occasional heartburn were all expressions of the building of the hot quality in her body.

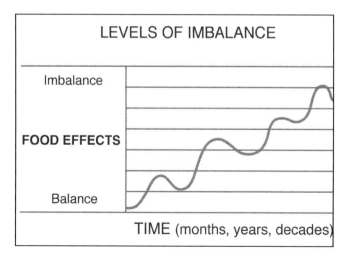

Notice this energy science model of healing says that you and I cause our disease because we are the unconscious choice makers urging ourselves out of balance. This is not about a "blame game" but rather empowering you to become a conscious choicemaker that leads to balance by using energy science tools described later.

You can do things either unconsciously or consciously to reduce the buildup of these qualities so you will not be provoking at any given moment. For instance, if you were a

PV eating raw tomatoes and onion in a salsa with corn tortilla chips, this would become a provoking event because both foods are in the No column that I'll cover in Chapter 4.

But if you unconsciously put loads of **cooling** cilantro with this provoking food combination, there would be less of an unbalancing effect.

This small but incremental and cumulative episode might be dissipated if no further provoking choices were made over a period. But due to the future unconscious choices, it is likely more provocation of the energy patterns will ensue with similar choices as the days, weeks, months, and years go by. The good news is that if you become more conscious about the choices you are making, you can begin to prevent the earliest provocations and hence IC flares in the energy physiology.

From our bathtub analogy, increased qualities of Vata and Pitta come to reside either in the GI tract or in the urinary tract, producing symptoms of an IC flare. Many times IC patients have very early symptoms of IC long before they actually begin having regular flares of the disease. This may be seen as urinary tract infection (UTI) symptoms treated as an infection with resolution. In reality this is simply a provoked energy complex that precedes the onset of overt IC.

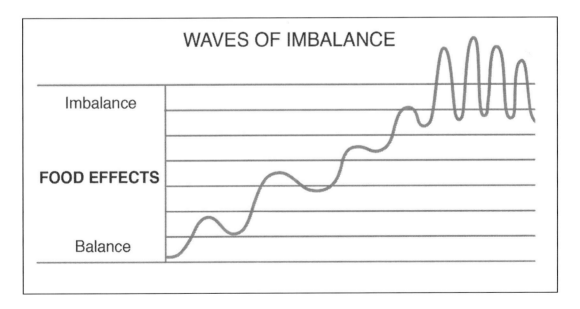

The above diagram depicts the final culmination of the imbalance where the symptoms of a UTI occur, but this time there is no relenting of symptoms. Wave after wave of flares begins, and visits to the doctor occur without symptom relief. Symptoms become intolerable and life becomes unmanageable.

Mary's Story

Mary now can remember her first UTI that seemed to start it all. The dates are not so important as the progression of the disease and the lack of ability to get help because the diagnosis was always a bacterial infection treated with antibiotics. Once she had a diagnosis of IC, the progression of her problem became clear. Now flares were seen as outward expressions of something not right in her body.

You begin having marital problems, difficulty at work with relationships, undue stress, and trouble sleeping. You find yourself going to the physician again for help. You have reached the top of the graph, where imbalance has led to intolerable imbalance and pain, which is the great motivator for change.

Your level of awareness in now such that you have the desire for change because you have encountered pain. And the physician will help direct that change by using pharmaceuticals to calm the matter field's molecular changes. **But you see now that these molecular changes being treated have deep, underlying energetic roots of imbalance.** And this imbalance over time takes a toll on the mindbody by depleting its energy stores through expending energy to maintain the disruption in the field itself.

The matter field physician may see this as an inflammatory condition. But the practitioner will see it as a molecular problem of excess acidity in the bladder and will use the potassium chloride sensitivity test to see if this is indeed IC. There is nothing wrong with this matter science approach. But it falls short of your ability to get to the root of the imbalance and certainly shackles you from dealing with it from a nutritional point of view.

Matter and Energy Science Contrast

Matter Science Medical Model	Energy Science Medical Model
Quantitative (by measurement)	Qualitative
Health is determined by provider	Health is a personal responsibility
Origin of disease is molecular	Origin of disease is quality imbalance
Disease is determined by labels	Disease is imbalance of VPK
Disease is treated by fixing molecules	Disease is treated by changing the imbalance of qualities

From an energy science approach, you will need much more work than taking a pharmaceutical if you intend to heal. Otherwise, anything short of this is a bandage. If a matter science nutritional approach is employed, it will be incomplete because it will miss significant foods that are triggering.

For example, who would find banana as inflammatory? But from the energy science view, the postdigestive effect of banana carries the qualities of the pungent and sour tastes leading to flares. This is one observation among hundreds demonstrating the power behind the energy science nutritional approach.

Because you are not doing everything wrong with respect to lifestyle choices, the time between these oscillating waves of imbalance can be quite drawn out. But nonetheless, they illustrate that imbalances do not go away but linger below the threshold only to show up later. What does this sine wave look like in day-to-day life?

You have good and bad days, good and bad weeks, good and bad months. You have periods where you feel tip-top and periods where you are not so good emotionally, physically, or both. These peaks of off days, weeks, or months are energetically manifested imbalances, and when the symptoms become intolerable, you take yourself to the doctor.

The important observation here is that even though you feel good, in reality you are just waiting for the next unpredictable wave flare to hit. No healing is occurring because the energetic imbalance that created the problem in the first place has not been addressed. If there are no abnormal molecular tests or measurements and the biopsies are negative, then obviously there is nothing wrong with your matter field and the doctor is correct.

There is nothing measurably wrong with the **gross** matter field. The problem lies in the energy field that is **subtly** manifesting as symptoms into the matter field, like a child crying for attention. But the attention does not come from taking a pill but by changing lifestyle behavior patterns that cause the imbalance leading to IC.

Matter Science Disease Labeling and Real Healing

In the matter science method of healing, disease labels are important in order to know how to treat the problem. There are broad categories such as autoimmune disorders and infectious diseases and then very specific names such as IC or breast cancer.

The danger with such a method is the built-in implication that if you rid your-self of the disease label then you return to health. As in the preceding description of the origins and progression of disease from an energy science model, this is usually not true. If you have breast cancer and have it removed, then the underlying imbalance that produced the breast cancer in the first place is still operative.

So when treating a disease label such as IC, if you embark on an energy science approach to deal with it, know that you are not only clearing IC but undergoing real healing. That is, you are clearing imbalances that led to the disease and therefore will clear the possibility of other diseases in the future. This kind of healing also supports how to head off imbalances at the level of the GI tract so that true prevention of disease is possible.

Inflammation and Disease Labeling

The concept of inflammation in the energy science medical discipline has been understood in terms of the **hot** quality, which is the manifestation of the transformative energy pattern of Pitta. The matter science medical model is now beginning to understand that inflammation underscores many if not all diseases of the human physiology.

From Alzheimer's to all forms of cancer, both energy and matter science models are on the same page with respect to the origin of disease. It is just that the energy science model uses the GI tract as the origin of all imbalances, whereas the matter science struggles with the molecular study of disease. And it is not to say that one way is incorrect and the other correct.

It is a matter of perspective. But the one important differentiating factor between the two is that **because the energy science sees the origins of disease as an expression of imbalance,** it has the rather unique capability to deal with the many chronic diseases such as IC that the matter science cannot address. Being able to address the painful suffering of flares, destruction of relationships, and the associated other medical conditions, the energy science medical discipline becomes a major contributing force in the treatment and management of such inflammatory chronic diseases.

Chronic Prostatitis

IC has a brother soul mate in male chronic prostatitis. It often is as common in a urological practice as IC. Since it is an inflammatory prostate condition, its presenting symptoms are lower abdominal and/or perineal (between the legs) pain. It is often associated with the same urinary symptoms of IC, but there can also be pain with ejaculation.

It sets itself apart from acute prostatitis, which usually exhibits fever and chills and bacteria in the urine. But in the chronic prostatitis presentation, most often the prostatic secretions, like the cultures in women with IC, are negative. X-ray workup or cystoscopy rarely reveals anything abnormal unless there are other presenting historical features such as blood in the urine.

It is not surprising that chronic prostatitis responds to antibiotics, and you now know why since antibiotics are in essence anti-inflammatory (reduces the energy pattern of Pitta). And antibiotics become the most common way of treating the condition.

GERD

This condition is the end stage of acid indigestion or hyperacidity (excess stomach acid). Simply put, too much acid formation in the stomach (excess **hot** quality or too much Pitta) affects the valve at the junction between the esophagus (tube from the mouth that delivers food to stomach) and the stomach. This valve does not function well due to the inflammatory swelling.

The stomach acid goes into the esophagus and leads to heartburn (notice that the term tells us that the **hot** quality is present). The link to nutrition is not widely accepted amongst gastroenterologists, and I would say the majority of these specialists use blocking drugs to deal with the problem. This is not to say there are not GI specialists who use nutrition as therapy, but from my experience it is unusual.

It comes as no surprise that the **hot** quality in the stomach and GI tract would not reach the general circulation and have to be eliminated by the urinary system, hence leading to IC flares. So currently the IC community discusses Prelief as an over-the-counter antacid to treat this associated disease label.

IBS

It is estimated that irritable bowel syndrome as a disease label is associated with IC 50 percent of the time. My clinical bias is that it is almost 100 percent of the time. This is because almost all disseminated energetic disease is associated with some form of bowel dysfunction, and IBS fits the bill. It is just that the condition does not show a broad enough group of symptoms to get the disease label.

Every disease in the human physiology as we know it has a spectrum of presentation. Some IBS can be very mild, while some people are incapacitated by the symptoms. The **hot** quality is involved here as well, which again is not surprising due to its IC association, and it leads to the diarrhea of IBS. The small intestine becomes irritable due to the **hot** and **mobile** qualities.

But the characteristic that sets IBS apart from other GI disease labels is its aspect of constipation. As I have discussed earlier, the hallmark of Vata aggravation in the GI tract results in colonic dysfunction and leads to slowing of colonic evacuation. The reason is that gas distends and fills the lower rectum, rendering the lining **dry, rough,** and **cold** hence ineffective in stool elimination due to primarily **dryness.**

Fibromyalgia

This inflammatory condition has a high association with IC and is marked by chronic widespread pain, fatigue, and heightened pain in response to pressure. As with most chronic inflammatory diseases, sleep disturbances are common. Palpitations often occur, and a Holter monitor is used to see if there are serious heart rhythm disturbances.

The qualities leading to IC in the urinary tract are increased throughout the body and so it is not surprising that the qualities could affect the muscle layer of the body leading to the symptoms of fibromyalgia.

IC and the aforementioned disease labels all have inflammation as the common pathway. From an energy science view, these are all treatable conditions. These will be treated separately in the continued book series.

Energy Science Long-Term IC Solution

As you saw in Mary's situation, IC can have its ups and downs. Alternative therapies may work for a while, but from an energy science medical view, unless the imbalances are addressed, then the energy patterns that brought about the IC in the first place will merely become less in their expression but not resolve.

It is important to continue to clear all symptoms of IC because the symptoms, even though less, still indicate that the imbalance of the involved qualities is present. You see, if these qualities are still in excess, then there is the real possibility of involvement of other organ systems that lead to other expressions of imbalance, such as fibromyalgia.

And this does not require focused attention after you have been doing the lifestyle energy science work. And it does not mean that if you eat the wrong thing that there is a major setback. The body slowly lets go of the unbalancing qualities. If you do the work and then step back and get out of the way, clearing of IC will be the final result.

Chapter Summary

The energy science of Ayurveda states that Nature is composed of ten pairs of vibrational frequencies or opposing qualities (e.g., hot and cold). You are part of Nature, and therefore you have these same opposing qualities. The energy science gives you tools to maintain balance of these qualities.

Any chronic disease is an imbalance of qualities. IC flares are waves of expressed excessive qualities in the urinary tract. The primary source of unbalancing qualities is the food you ingest. Foods deliver the qualities that become excessive, although these qualities may come from other activities and the environment as well.

This energy science model of Ayurveda says that you and I cause our disease because we are the unconscious choice makers throwing ourselves out of balance. This is not a "blame game" here but rather an effort to empower us into being conscious rather than unconscious choice makers, people who are conscious of choices that lead to balance with Nature by using energy science tools.

The qualities of **light, cold, rough, dry, mobile, sharp, hot, liquid,** and **spreading** are responsible for the inflammatory symptoms of IC when they are excessively expressed in the urinary tract. These same qualities can be expressed in the GI tract, producing IBS and GERD, and in the muscular system, producing fibromyalgia.

IC is a debilitating noninfectious inflammatory condition of the bladder that is composed of several energetically related Pitta-provoked disease states or labels. This syndrome includes chronic prostatitis in men, irritable bowel syndrome (IBS), gastroesophageal reflux disease (GERD), and fibromyalgia.

Next I'll talk about the energy patterns of Vata, Pitta, and Kapha that I've referred to previously.

Chapter 3

Seeing Interstitial Cystitis in a Different Way

"There is no escape from IC. It's there every morning to greet my day. It invades every area of my life. My marriage, friendships, children, all my relationships. My sanity. It is an invisible enemy, as I look great on the outside but suffer unbearably at times on the inside. Which of course no one can see."

In the energy science medical tradition, balance brings about health. For example, the anger and frustration that you feel about IC are expressions of the very imbalance of the **hot** quality that is causing your chronic disease. Eventually your energy is drained and you are left emotionally sad, despondent, and depressed.

If there is too much **hot** and **mobile** qualities localized in the urinary tract, then IC can be the result. And this experience of the **hot** quality may not show up as feeling excessively **hot**, but expressed as intense appetite, diarrhea, need for **cold** iced drinks, sudden temper outbursts, and blaming others for your problems.

You also learned that these **qualities make up everything in Nature,** including yourself as a biologic energy field as well as the foods that you eat. So too much **hot** quality in the food can increase the existing **hot** quality in the body. This is the essence of seeing how foods create disease. In the energy science biological world, it is not the molecule that causes disease but rather the choices that produce the imbalance of qualities in your body.

If you have IC and unknowingly eat foods that carry the **hot** and **mobile** qualities, you are likely playing with fire and a flare. However, it is difficult for you to understand how these qualities play out in yourself, so there is another layer that can be useful in helping us see the body as an energy field. These are called energy patterns. This layer is an excellent tool for witnessing yourself when active in your chronic disease of IC. Let's explore this layer in more detail.

Mindbody Energy Patterns

The ten pairs of qualities organize to form the energy patterns of Vata, Pitta, and Kapha (VPK). These are true psychophysiologic (mindbody) expressions in that they are physically and mentally expressed, and by using the tools to create balance you bring these energy patterns into balance. As you will experience, seeing yourself as energy patterns is a profound way to begin witnessing or seeing yourself in action (the "there I go again" moment of observing).

Vata is the pattern of movement. Anything that happens in the mindbody involved with movement is the energy pattern of Vata at work. The movement of blood, food, and thought are all aspects of Vata. It is the least physically expressed of the energy patterns and is closest to the workings of the nervous system, mind and the energy field. The qualities associated with this pattern are **light, cold, rough, dry, subtle, mobile,** and **clear**.

Pitta is the energy pattern of transformation. Anything that happens in the mindbody involved with change of form is Pitta at work. The change of ingested broccoli into heart and lung cells is an aspect of Pitta. Digestion of ideas, beliefs, and emotions are transformative tasks of Pitta as well. The unique qualities of Pitta are **light, sharp, hot, oily, liquid,** and **spreading.**

Kapha is the pattern of stability and is the most physically expressed in contrast to Vata. It stabilizes and grounds the mindbody. It has the most qualities associated with it due to its material expression. The qualities are **heavy, dull, cold, smooth, oily, dense, liquid, hard, soft, gross, static,** and **cloudy.**

For your purposes, the most important qualities to remember is that Vata is **light, cold, rough, dry,** and **mobile;** Pitta is **sharp, hot, liquid,** and **spreading; and** Kapha is **heavy, dull, cool,** and **static.** Notice that Pitta is the only energy pattern that has the **hot** quality. This will be important to remember as you read along.

Energy Patterns: Balanced and Unbalanced

Vata

Individuals with Vata predominance (ectomorph) when in balance are thin with a small degree of muscle mass indicative of the **light** quality. They have quick minds (**mobile**) but poor memory and are highly creative. Variable appetite and eating patterns mark their nutritional habits. They prefer to snack rather than eat a full meal.

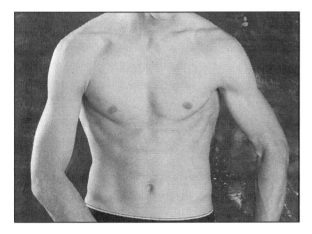

When out of balance, they have a tendency to become scattered without focus. In regards to bowels, people with Vata predominance become constipated. Because Vata's principle elements are space and air, there can be excessive passage of gas or flatus. They become flighty and anxious with a tendency to a fast paced lifestyle. They are prone to osteoporosis due to the **light** quality in the bone structure. They have difficulty gaining or keeping weight due to the irregular eating pattern. The typical coping strategy is to run away.

If you have a high Vata predominance, you have the chance of being pushed over the top, and this can lead to other Vata disorders, such as chronic fatigue syndrome, adrenal fatigue, and fibromyalgia. An Ayurvedic axiom says, "Treat Vata like a flower, Pitta like your best friend, and Kapha like your enemy." Each of these energy patterns has its strengths and weaknesses.

Vata loves to move but doesn't have the endurance and stamina to keep it up for long (sprinter versus long-distance runner). Hence Vata-predominant patients have the likelihood of overdoing and exhausting themselves. This is an important point that Vata-predominant people need to learn over and over again in their lifetimes.

Keep in mind that even though the pictures depict the matter field expressions of these energy patterns, they also convey the way these energy patterns think and behave in the world—that is, the energy patterns are psychological expressions as well.

Pitta

Individuals with Pitta predominance have modest body builds (mesomorph) and, often, reddish hair and/or complexions indicating the **hot** quality. They have a strong appetite, and intellectually they are intense and disciplined. Their favorite phrases are "interesting" and "I see," indicating their visual strength.

When out of balance, Pitta-predominant people become inflamed. Their skin may become red due to excess heat on the surface of the skin. The bowels of Pitta-predominant individuals will produce diarrhea. They can gain weight easily due to the intense appetite. Anger, impatience, and easy frustration are hallmark imbalanced emotions. They tend to want to control everything and easily blame and react with a tendency toward "picking" on everything.

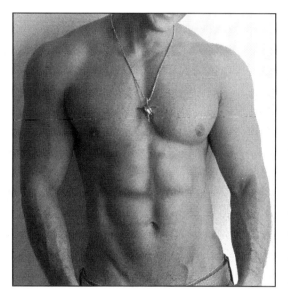

Psychologically, Pitta's **hot** quality brings intensity, focus, and drive. These mental qualities enable Pitta-dominant people to be highly competitive, which may burn up the Pitta dominant person due to the overexpressed **hot** quality. Mentally, when high, a Pitta-dominant person becomes judgmental, critical, and rigid. Rather than entertaining new, creative ways of doing things, there is a tendency to stonewall new possibilities, which can stand in the way of healing or improving relationships.

When out of balance, Pitta tends to overdo everything because of its intensity. Because of this, fatigue and exhaustion occurs from overdoing due to focus, in contrast with Vata, whose fatigue is due to lack of stamina and endurance. Pitta's coping strategy is to fight, while Vata's strategy is flight or run away.

Kapha

The most physically expressed of the energy patterns is Kapha (endomorph), who is thick in physical presentation. Kapha-predominant people are very attractive have a luster to their skin and age gracefully. They are strong, with great stamina and endurance. They have slow digestion and appetite. Mentally they process slowly but have a very good memory. They get along with everyone.

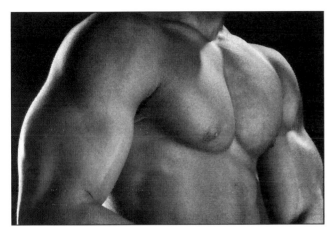

When out of balance, Kapha is prone to emotional eating and favors cookies, candy, and chocolate. Kapha's problems are inertia, procrastination, congestion, and weight gain. Due to the strong sense channels of taste and smell, a Kapha-dominant person's favorite pastime is to eat and enjoy the pleasures of the sensory experience. Coupled with slow metabolism, this makes weight gain a problem. The control drama is passivity, hoping problems will go away.

As you will see with the other energy patterns, Pitta-dominant individuals are prone to irritability, impatience, and anger, so you'd like to stay on their good side and not rile them. Kapha has trouble with inertia, so lighting a fire under Kapha individuals is at times necessary for them to get off point zero. When Kapha dominance is present, you have to push on this energy pattern to get it going. *Move* becomes the order of the day.

Most people express two energy patterns as dominant, although at times one of the energy patterns of Vata, Pitta, and Kapha can dominate over the other two, but this is unusual. The best way to determine the energy body makeup of an individual is to feel the pulse, since these energy patterns are physiologically expressed in the body. But at times this is not possible, the next best thing is to take a questionnaire, as in the appendix.

Be aware this at times can be misleading, but my experience has been that it is close enough to steer you in the right direction of the correct nutritional format. The combinations of PV, PK, or VK are expressed as being codominant. Nutritional formats, as you will see, are shown as two dominant energy patterns.

If you go to the appendix, you can take a test that will help determine your energy makeup and from there you can determine the nutritional format to follow.

IC and the Energy Patterns

IC is a Vata/Pitta disorder. The qualities of Vata and Pitta are expressed in excess or in an unbalanced way in the pelvis. Let's see how this works.

What happens when you have a flare? The **mobile, dry,** and **rough** quality of Vata is expressed in urinary frequency. The urgency or intensity of the need for urination is Pitta expressed in the **sharp** and **spreading** qualities.

The burning in the bladder, pelvic, vaginal, and rectal areas are related to the **hot, liquid,** and **spreading** qualities of Pitta. The maintenance of this unbalanced state in the pelvis is due to the **light** and **mobile** qualities of Vata because it moves Pitta to the pelvic site, where symptoms occur.

Kapha may be involved but secondarily. Because of the overweight condition, the **hot** quality of Pitta may become overexpressed due to the insulative nature of Kapha and subcutaneous fat.

> *Mary's Story*
> *Throughout her early life, Mary was thin. After her kids she continued to have the problem gaining weight, but it wasn't as bad. But as she began having the flares and diarrhea from IBS, she noticed a stronger appetite. She was now more aware of irritability and easy frustration around even small things. And her anxiety about IC and what the future had in store for her would set off a flare.*

Seeing the Body as an Energy Field

The value of the VPK paradigm is you now begin seeing yourself not as a collection of molecules but with a deeper reality, i.e., as a **subtle** energy field. This paradigm is an invitation, and there are several advantages.

Using VPK allows you to witness better. Does that sound strange? Witnessing is that state when you say to yourself, "There I go again." It is the state of observing yourself in action.

This witnessing state has many different terms associated with it. *Awareness* and *mindfulness* are those that are used frequently. Whatever you call it, the key is that witnessing produces health. Many productive, successful people use it as a tool, but others not at all.

It is only when you can observe present habits, place them up to energy science guidelines, and make changes that health can be achieved. **But who says that these guidelines are the ones to follow?**

The energy science of Ayurveda states that Nature herself sets the guidelines through the expressed qualities. For example, all of Nature takes its biggest meal at noon to take advantage of the strength of digestion (**hot**) at that time; Nature goes to bed (**static**) between nine and eleven at night (it is known that night-shift working is not conducive to good health); Nature becomes quiet just before sunrise and sunset (best time to quiet the mind through meditation).

The knowledge of VPK helps you observe yourself because you have a reference point when you are in and out of balance. You know what it looks like when you are healthy and what you look like when you are not. You know that fatigue associated with IC is not normal, so doing energy science work can give you back your stamina and endurance.

For example, if Pitta/Kapha (PK) has symptoms of IC, the **hot** quality can be brought about by the overweight condition. **So PKs should focus on losing weight to heal their IC as part of their strategy. All the aloe in the world will not deal with IC if a PK does not lose weight.**

Another benefit of the VPK energy paradigm is that the observations tend to reduce victimhood. You become empowered. There is great value in distancing yourself from the imbalance and laying off the problem to IC. When PV or PK is out of balance, then you know what to do rather than feeling hapless and helpless about the disease, which is what happens when the matter science approach is used.

IC and the Energy Patterns

Pitta is the only energy pattern that has the **hot** quality, and because of this it is the energy of transformation and metabolism of the body. When this energy localizes outside the GI tract, it produces searing, **sharp**, and **penetrating** pain.

This is the pain of IC. Burning on urination mimics a urinary tract infection. This burning occurs in the bladder, vagina, and even rectum when the Pitta qualities are high.

But whenever the Pitta and Kapha energy patterns leave the GI tract, they are carried by Vata, which is the only energy pattern that has the **mobile** quality. So if Pitta is present in the pelvis, then the Vata energy pattern is there as well.

The Vata qualities of **light, mobile, dry,** and **rough** lead to the urinary symptoms of urgency, frequency, and the feeling of incomplete emptying of the bladder. Although the **hot** quality of Pitta causes bladder wall irritability and reduced bladder capacity, it is Vata's presence that produces the disruption in voiding pattern.

So from an energy science view, IC is a Vata Pitta imbalance and needs to be treated as such. However, the person being treated must be taken into consideration. A PV patient will have subtle differences in management compared with a PK patient.

Overactive Bladder and IC

The disease label of the overactive bladder (OAB) is different from IC since it does not have the Pitta inflammatory component leading to the burning and severe pain. However, it does have the frequency, urgency, and feeling of incomplete bladder emptying associated with IC. It is actually a Vata imbalance without the Pitta component.

Because of this, OAB should be treated differently than IC, since energetically it is not at all like IC. Urologists can confuse it with neurogenic disease, but it's hard for the matter science to justify a disease label of neurological origin in an otherwise healthy woman in her twenties or thirties. So a new disease label of OAB was made for this particular group of patients, since they do not fit the label of IC.

The Concept of Release

Once the urinary tract is involved with the energy patterns of Vata and Pitta, the symptoms of Vata presence begin episodic expression of **light, cold**, **rough**, **dry,** and **mobile,** which lead to urgency, frequency, and a feeling of incomplete emptying of the bladder. Pitta's presence of inflammation leads to burning on urination and burning pain in the pelvis, vagina, and even rectum due to the **sharp**, **hot, liquid,** and **spreading** qualities.

These qualities lodge in the urinary tract and express as energy or wave. If you remember, the body as a matter field expresses itself as a particle or molecule. But as an energy field, the body shows wave-like patterns of change. So the intermittent flares that occur in the body are waves of energy and an expression of imbalance.

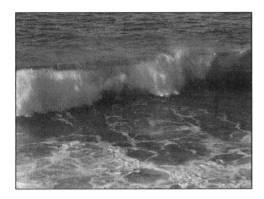

But what happens when you decide to do things differently? You begin paying attention to your day and how you live it. Nutrition becomes important, and you start seeing food as medicine. You choose certain foods and herbs that can help reduce the **hot** and **mobile** qualities of IC, and you use them regularly.

When you no longer support the overexpression of these qualities in the body by the foods that you eat, the body naturally begins letting go of these excess qualities of **light, cold**, **rough**, **dry, mobile, sharp**, **hot, liquid,** and **spreading.** This takes time, but by and by there is lessening of the symptoms that the qualities brought, and healing begins to occur.

What you see is gradual regression of the symptoms, not cessation. Symptoms diminish in a wave-like fashion, and there is a recession of the complex of symptoms, much like the outgoing tide on the beach. **This is a very important insight because if you don't understand the continued but lessened complex of flares, you may feel that what you are doing is not being effective.**

Curable Not Just Treatable Requires Radical Transformation

Those with IC are told by matter science physicians that the condition is treatable but not curable. This is unfortunate because it gives you a mind-set that there is nothing left for you to do but quietly suffer and garner support from online threads or your local support group. But as you have seen, the energy science states, "Clear the imbalance of qualities, clear the disease."

Hopefully this breath of fresh air changes the mind-set and clears the mind to produce clarity rather than despondency, haplessness, and hopelessness. Yes, it requires effort, discipline, and determination. In the words of an experienced Ayurvedic practitioner, it's possible to cure IC but it requires dedication and guidance, which will lead to a radical transformation that will produce an incredible state of health far from what you could imagine.

But in the end, you will achieve what you want: a pain-free life of freedom to do what you need to do without restrictions. And by the accompanying graph,

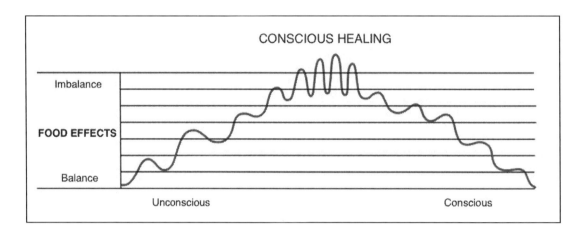

it's not as if this happens overnight. Month by month by doing energy work, you reach new levels of balance and health not achieved before. So as you progress you will have better states of health with mild lingering symptoms but nothing like what you're experiencing now.

The reason I can be so confident in making this curable statement is because of my own experience and that of many others whom I have chaperoned through the process of dealing with their IC. It is possible. You just have to get rid of the negative mind-set that this disease is not curable and stick to the energy science work necessary to begin the healing process.

How Long Does It Take to Start Feeling Better?

As I have just outlined, the lifestyle energy science changes are geared to reverse the physiologic imbalances leading to the IC complex of symptoms. As there are multiple ways to go out of balance over time, there are multiple ways to create balance. Indeed, it is not about just one or two things that bring about balance but a multiplicity of lifestyle measures.

Initially what energy science healing requires is the choice of doing things different-

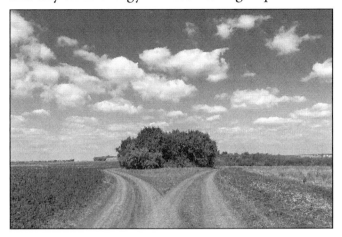

ly. You have been on one path determined by what you have been told. Now you have a different choice.

You can recognize by the preceding graphs that symptoms ramp up to the point where unpredictable flares become a way of life. This energetic imbalance is not created overnight but rather over months, years, and in some cases decades. So it will take time to reverse these unbalancing lifestyle choices.

In 2003, a retrospective study was done in my office of forty-five patients with IC. Ninety-one percent of these patients had a 50 percent or more reduction in their symptoms with the Pitta nutritional format and aloe vera gel. The complete summary of this study can be found at http://bit.ly/OQSVz1. This gives you a glimpse of what to expect, but everyone is unique with respect to the individual's imbalance and length of disease.

This paper was read at the NW Urology Society in 2005 and was almost published in the *Journal of the Canadian Urological Association.* It had undergone a thorough committee review and was set for publication in its final galley print when someone got **cold** feet and pulled the article without explanation to me. I guess it was just too much for mainstream matter science to handle.

Timeline for Healing IC

As a child you may have asked, "Are we there yet?" So when will this IC be over? Obviously, this is a common question. The short answer is, "It's over when it's over." But to be more specific, in general **it takes two months of release for every year of imbalance**. So if you have had symptoms of IC for ten years, it will take twenty months of work to clear the abnormal energy complex.

Would you not find it hard to believe if an athlete showed up for matches without training or preparation? You know that in life there is nothing for free. You know that whatever you obtain in life comes with effort and determination.

Health is a skill that you get better at. It's not something you hope for, but it's something you get by doing work toward that end. The energy science of Ayurveda gives you the tools to get the skill of health.

You have been trained to believe that if you want health you take yourself to the doctor, who deems you are healthy because your blood pressure and blood tests are normal. But from an energy science perspective, health is determined not by the doctor but by how you feel. You just have to pay attention.

So health becomes our personal responsibility. Healing IC is that way, and having ongoing health is the same way.

Chapter Summary

The qualities organize to form the energy patterns of Vata, Pitta, and Kapha (VPK). The energy pattern of movement is Vata, Pitta is the energy of transformation, and Kapha is the energy of stability. In order to function as an energy field, you need all three patterns.

Each of us has different proportions of these energy patterns, and typically two of the three are dominantly expressed. Those that dominate usually lead us to disease. When these energy patterns are in balance, there is no disharmony or disease.

But when the qualities that are associated with the energy patterns become excessive, imbalance occurs and so does disease. For example, if you are Vata (V) and Pitta (P) dominant and IC is a VP disease, then IC is possible.

When you pay attention by witnessing behavior patterns, then release of excessive qualities that have accumulated is possible. Then healing is a real possibility. Ninety-one percent of people using a Pitta nutritional format and aloe vera gel see a 50 percent reduction in symptoms in six weeks. But for complete resolution of IC, it will take two months of energy work for every year since the beginning of symptoms.

So let's explore the energy science's view of balanced nutrition.

Chapter 4

Producing Balance Through Foods

"One caveat: Diet in IC is a very individual thing. When I read the list of foods that were deemed to be safe for IC, my reaction to the inclusion of some of them was 'I wish I could eat that!'"

It is well-known that food choice is important in the management of IC and, as a matter of fact, all chronic disease. As you have read, the easiest way to cause an IC flare is to eat foods that produce an imbalance in yourself. This is because the qualities in the food increase the qualities in your own physiology, usually resulting in the excess **hot** quality of inflammation.

The current molecular science approach to diet has no ability to relate the physiological consequences of food to us personally. What is good for one person is not good for another, and you know by personal experience that this is the case. This diet approach pales in comparison with the more comprehensive energy science nutrition, which is based on a philosophy about the conscious workings of Nature Herself, not on molecular observations, mythology, and guesswork.

One of the most important gifts of energy science nutrition is that ingested foods need to be tailored to individual energy patterns. Someone with IC and a strong Pitta imbalance with a lot of the **hot** quality already is much more easily provoked with foods carrying the **hot** quality than a person with a Vata- or Kapha-dominant makeups who have the **cold** quality. This sets the Ayurvedic nutritional approach apart from the current Western diet approach and is a salient contribution to nutritional management of disease.

Nutrition Facts

Serving Size 1 Bar (85g)
Servings Per Container 4

Amount Per Serving

Calories 170	Calories from Fat 50

% Daily Value *

Total Fat 6g	**9%**
Saturated Fat 4g	**19%**
Trans Fat 0g	
Polyunsaturated Fat 0.5g	
Monounsaturated Fat 1g	
Cholesterol 13mg	**4%**
Sodium 83mg	**3%**
Total Carbohydrate 33g	**11%**
Dietary Fiber 4g	**16%**
Sugar 25g	
Protein 3g	

Vitamin A 110%	•	Vitamin C 2%	
Calcium 10%	•	Iron 3%	

*Percent Daily Values are based on a 2,000 calorie diet. Your daily values may be higher or lower depending on your calorie needs.

	Calories	2,000	2,500
Total Fat	Less than	65g	80g
Sat Fat	Less than	20g	25g
Cholesterol	Less than	300mg	300mg
Sodium	Less than	2,400mg	2,400mg
Total Carbohydrate		300g	375g
Dietary Fiber		25g	30g

Calories per gram:
Fat 9 • Carbohydrate 4 • Protein 4

It also explains why the molecular approach has failed the health-conscious consumer. The energy science approach explains to you why bananas are inflammatory, why fast foods can be balancing for Vata but a terrible choice for Kapha (and not based on fat content), and why our love affair with the tomato is problematic.

As mentioned earlier the energetic qualities are intellectual concepts until you begin to associate them with the energy body experience. It requires reframing your observations. Heartburn, a bladder flare, or diarrhea are symptoms of the **hot** quality. When you begin to reframe you observations in terms of the energy body then the energy body is not an intellectual concept but a real tangible experience.

Trigger Foods

The matter science dietary approach to IC is to determine personal trigger foods. The elimination diet has been used for decades to help determine possible food allergies and has been used with some success in the IC community. But this approach is hit or miss and makes it difficult to be sure what foods carry the offending "molecules" or effects. In the end it becomes virtual guesswork except for the obvious choices such as white chicken (good), refined sugar (bad), or coffee(bad).

The difficulty with this approach is twofold. First a flare may occur, but it is problematic to find which food was the offending agent. This leads to a second problem, which is the danger of walking yourself into a "dietary corner." Literally, food choices begin to be sectored away from the mainstream of choices, such that nothing is safe anymore, particularly when the flares are extremely painful.

Other problems with this approach are the need for excessive dietary diary entries and the possibility of interpreting foods that produce "an allergic reaction." In the end, the matter science diet approach is not very effective for chronic disease.

The GI Tract as Cause of Disease

The gastrointestinal (GI) tract from an energy science view is the source of the excessive qualities that occur from foods ingested. The qualities build up over time and may produce GI symptoms such as GERD or IBS. Eventually these qualities leave the GI tract and lodge in certain areas that are predisposed to receiving them.

The central role of the GI tract in the disease process of the energy science model cannot be emphasized enough. This is why diet has become such a foundational piece in the matter science management of IC as espoused by the IC support groups in the United States. A patient who held the consensus belief that molecules cause disease and not our choices told me, "I can't believe foods were responsible for my symptoms."

There is a natural propensity for excess acidity in the form of the **hot** quality to seek elimination through the urine, as the kidneys are responsible for acid base balance. Hence acid loading (increased expression of the Pitta energy pattern) in the GI tract can lead to acid loading in the urinary tract, hence predisposing the latter to IC.

When the excess **hot** quality is maintained in the GI tract over time, it begins to aggravate the gut muscle to the point of irritability and increased motility. You recognize this excess **mobility** as diarrhea because the transit time in the gut doesn't allow enough water to be removed from the bowel contents, and diarrhea is the result. When this becomes a chronic condition, it becomes labeled as IBS.

As the **hot** quality becomes excessive in the body, inflammation is the end result. This inflammatory picture is seen in many different organ systems but the source is always the same, the GI tract. Inflammation is now being associated with almost all diseases in the matter science realm, indicating the prevalence of the Pitta energy pattern of transformation in the disease process.

Removal of Guesswork

Using an energy science nutritional approach for food choices removes food diaries and is elegant in its simplicity. Just follow the list at icdiet.com, and you're done! Or if you want a more refined approach with more choices, you can take the test at foodsheal.com. Or go to the appendix of this book and use the appropriate nutritional format for your mindbody energy makeup.

Our current matter science nutritional information is not a system, but rather a collection of data about the foods we ingest. You may know a lot about broccoli, the number of calories per gram, the number of carbohydrates per gram, and the vitamin and mineral content, but this quantitative analysis cannot tell me if broccoli resonates with *my* physiology. I just know a lot about broccoli quantitatively.

The energy science approach is based on a philosophy about the conscious workings of Nature herself, not on errant molecular observations, mythology, and guesswork. When you ingest foods, you are ingesting Nature's universal qualities that you are as well.

Because of this, the energy makeup of the individual dictates food choices. If you have the **hot** quality in inflammatory excess, then taking in more of that quality produces an imbalance and potentially a flare. This is a salient observation that sets apart the matter and energy science approaches to disease.

Nutrition Versus Diet

But the energy science approach goes even further. It takes "diet" to a new science of understanding. Whether you know it or not, you are looking for a nutritional approach to foods, something that will bring sanity to a confused discipline. "I eat healthy" is a common refrain but has virtually no meaning. The individual defines healthy food choices based on worn-out belief systems that are often energetically incorrect.

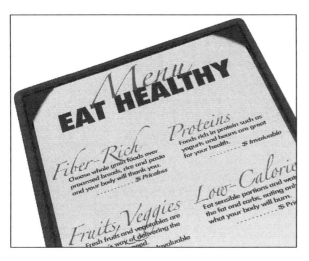

Whether corn is organic, the vegetable is raw, the meat is buffalo, or the fast food is nutritious, the food must resonate with your own individual physiology for it to be healthy. So you shouldn't be eating corn, even if organic, if it doesn't resonate with you.

A nutritional system goes beyond diet because it takes into account among other things appetite or digestive fire (more about that in chapter five), incompatible food combinations, bowel activity or the lack thereof, and the psychological effects of food. Nutrition should be much more than the measurement of molecules you ingest.

Diet	Nutrition
Molecule basis	Energy basis
Quantitative	Qualitative
No philosophical pinnings	Aligned with functions of Nature
Group basis	Individual basis
No incompatible food combinations	Incompatible food combining
Health is the absence of disease	Evaluates GI function with relationship to food
Consumer confusion	Consumer clarity
Involves evaluation of food	Involves all bodily processes around food

When you participate in nutrition, balance automatically happens. If you step out of the way and become quiet (another way of saying slow down the thoughts) and do energetic nutritional work, the mindbody will naturally seek the balance that Nature intended. Diet disengages us from Nature, and nutrition makes us one with Nature. There's nothing wrong with studying the action of molecules on the mindbody, but don't rely just on that information to afford you health.

Lastly our current obsession with weight gain has amplified this matter science approach to foods even more because you become a calorie counter and obsessed with the molecular effects of food. But the problem with the approach is that looking at foods in this way does not tell you how specific foods affect you.

Rhythms of Nature

Try to step out of Nature, right now. Go ahead, see if you can do it. I'll wait right here. Physically or mentally or both, get out of here (Nature). Not possible? Yes, that's right. As a matter of fact, it's mission impossible!

You are intimately associated with all that is around you, and the energy patterns of Vata, Pitta, and Kapha are aspects or faces of Nature. We observe Kapha dogs, Vata hummingbirds, and Pitta lions. These energy patterns are also involved in how we view time.

Between 6 a.m. and 10 a.m. is a Kapha time, a **heavy, cold,** and **slow/dull** time, so it's not such a good idea to have a heavy breakfast unless you plan a lot of activity to overcome these qualities. Between 10 a.m. and 2 p.m. is a Pitta time, where the qualities of **hot** and **sharp/penetrating** are expressed, so this is the best time for the day's biggest meal. Between 2 p.m. and 6 p.m. is a Vata time, with the **cold, light** and **mobile** qualities. This is great time for activity.

Between 6 p.m. and 10 p.m. is another **heavy, cold, slow/dull** time, so it's not a good time for a heavy meal but time for winding down. Between 10 p.m. and 2 a.m. is another period where the **hot, sharp/penetrating** qualities are being used for body detoxification. Between 2 a.m. and 6 a.m. is another Vata period, where the qualities of **cold, light, mobile** are expressed, and this is the time for emotional detoxification during dream states.

These qualities that are bolded are most prominent in Nature's physiology, but you mirror them yourself physiologically as well. Do you notice that you are hungry around noontime and late at night? Do you eat breakfast at times when you are really not hungry? Do you feel sharpest in the afternoon when working on projects? Do you find that it's hard getting started in the morning and that the evening is a great time to wind down from the day?

Taste as Causation of IC Flares

Since you are part of Nature, you have energetically the same qualities as the foods you consume. When you ingest foods, you are ingesting Nature, and you sense these aspects of Nature as a group of qualities that are called tastes—for example, the salty taste that you may recognize on the tongue as sensations of **hot, heavy, oily,** and **liquid** qualities that are pervasive throughout Nature, including yourself as an energy field.

Since salty has the **hot** quality, it could potentiate an IC flare. Likewise the tastes of sour and pungent can provoke Pitta due to the **hot** and **sharp** qualities respectively. So the tastes of sour, salty, and pungent can provoke your IC. Hence the root causes of IC are the nutritional choices that you make on a chronic basis for many years. The good news is that by simply avoiding these tastes, you can reverse the process.

The balancing tastes for IC are sweet, bitter, and astringent. These tastes bring on the **cold** quality of foods. However, this actually becomes impossible to figure out on your own. So how can you figure out whether broccoli is good or bad for you?

The Good News: Nutritional Formats

I have taken you through the reasons why foods are classified as they are in the energy science, but as you can see, complexity develops quickly. The good news is that there are nutritional formats that can be used to guide you along the way. These are located in the appendix, as is a questionnaire to help determine your mindbody energy makeup.

After determining your mindbody makeup—VP, KP, or VK—then simply go to the appropriate format and you can now make balancing food choices around foods that will not produce imbalance and allow your mindbody to heal IC. Each format has Yes, No, and Moderation columns. The latter would be consumed two or three times per week, and a preferred way of looking at this column is to dance in and out of it. The Yes column becomes the primary staple of food choice.

The purpose of these food lists is to give guidance, not rules. The mindbody rebels at being told no to anything, so be easy with this information. But realize that there is great wisdom here, and if applied gradually over a three-month period, you can have changes in terms of frequency of flare and intensity.

There is never just one solution to any health problem with which you are confronted. The process will always require a multifaceted approach because that which caused the imbalance in the first place was multifaceted.

Solutions to No

Food choices in the No column do not mean never. If you go out to a friend's home for dinner and several items are served in the No column, you might honor your friend and eat the No items with awareness and interest as to what the physiological effects will be. It may be that there are no observable effects to your awareness, but it is clear from an energy perspective that these foods create imbalances in the energy physiology that over time will produce problems.

From an energy science perspective, foods are not inherently right or wrong, good or bad. The lists begin to help you witness that certain foods produce untoward physiologic consequences if you become deliberate about your observations. You can point to the fact that no one has died acutely because the person ate foods that were in the No column.

But many of us die a chronic death from chronic ingestion of foods that lead to severe imbalances. Use of No foods after two or three days will lead to a flare. As you become stronger and more in balance, these foods will not be as provoking, particularly if the digestive fire is strong (next chapter).

The key is taking baby steps with foods that are your favorites. In this way you can gradually cut back. Another possibility is to give yourself the taste without swallowing a large amount of the food. Or, for example, try substitutes for peanut butter by using sunflower butter.

Many have reported that when starting on a nutritional format that they felt like their life was over. Their freedom of choice had been taken from them and all of the "favs" were never to be tasted again. But something miraculous happens when you give the "friends" up.

You begin to find that they were cravings of the mind not based on bodily needs. Then it's easy to not go back. And if you go back and check it out, you do it with clarity of perception.

Food Incompatibility

The appendix also has a list of foods that are energetically incompatible with each other. These food-combining dictums are very important and act like the No list of the just-mentioned nutritional information. For example, freshly made yogurt can be safely eaten with rice, ghee, and toast but would be harmful with fruit, milk, cheese, eggs, meat, fish, nightshades, and hot drinks.

Or it would be a mistake to combine fruit with any other food. This is a central theme throughout the listing of the food incompatibility table and underscores the fact that the digestive fire or enzyme system of the gastrointestinal (GI) tract is adversely affected by using fruits as simple sugars with more complex carbohydrates, proteins, and fats.

The reason for this from a molecular standpoint is that simple sugars that are quickly broken down at the brush border of the gut mucosa interfere with the digestion, absorption, and assimilation of more complex carbohydrates, proteins, and fats. While eating an unbalancing combination once in a while will not cause adverse physiological problems, not adhering to them on a relatively consistent basis will lead to definite imbalance in the GI tract and the buildup of undigested debris.

This undigested material in the gut will eventually begin clogging the lymph channels, which in part are responsible for carrying away nutrients from the gut lumen.

Incompatible combination examples are eggs used with milk, cheese and meat, which becomes an omelet, and beans with cheese and meat, which is a taco. Potato does not combine with dairy, so milk with mashed potatoes or baked potatoes with sour cream or butter are problems. Honey should never be cooked because it acts like a sticky, gooey adhesive substance on the gut lining, which becomes toxic to the GI tract.

Dairy Products: Milk and Yogurt and Their Value with IC

Mother's milk is the complete food and contains all 6 tastes. But cow's milk is a difficult food to digest due to the size of the proteins that require digestive attention. Always heating milk before drinking it is a good idea and using spices with it enhances your ability to digest it. This is why chai is such a good drink to use because it uses spices with the milk to stoke digestion and at the same time brings the nutritious benefits of milk.

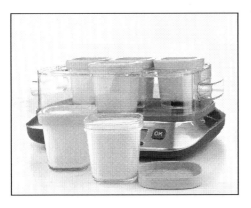

Yogurt should not be used with milk as this is a poor food combination. It is a predigested milk product with "good" bacteria for GI tract colonization which is a major contributor to digestive fire that I'll talk about in the next chapter.

From an energy science view yogurt that is bought in the store is not a healthy food and should be avoided. From an IC point of view this is because over time in storage yogurt becomes too acidic due to the low grade activity of the organisms in the product. For this reason the energy science recommends that if you are to use yogurt you should make your own, that is, home made yogurt.

Homemade yogurt can be made done very easily with commercially available yogurt makers purchased online or in stores. Remember to not use fruit with it as this is an acidic food combination.

Hard cheeses as dairy are aged and therefore acidic. Examples include cheddar, swiss, and parmesan. Soft cheeses such as gouda, mozzarella, and blue cheese are better less acidic choices. Another soft cheese alternative is paneer, a soft cheese that you can make yourself in the kitchen.

Specific Foods for IC

Since foods are medicine, you would expect that certain foods can be used very specifically for IC. Those foods, of course, would be **cool**ing to the body to reverse the inflammatory **hot** quality. This **cool**ing is not the type of **cool**ing that you're familiar with, such as when drinking a cold glass of water with ice cubes (not recommended, as it disturbs digestion).

The type of **cool**ing I'm referring to is energetic **cool**ing, which from an Ayurvedic point of view is the **subtle** effect that the foods have on the GI tract and simultaneously on the body. These **cool**ing effects of foods are enhanced by **cool**ing herbs that may be used with them.

This list is not exhaustive by any means and is limited only by your imagination and the nutritional formats provided for you.

Coconut Milk Smoothie

> 1 cup coconut milk
> 1 cup sweet strawberries, cherries, or other berries available in season
> 0.5 tsp Sucanat
> 1 tablespoon coconut flakes
> Blenderize and add water to change consistency.

Cucumber Milk

Cut up half of a cucumber and blenderize it with a cup of room-temperature cow's milk with half a teaspoon of cumin or turmeric. Milk acts as a taxicab to take the **cool**ing qualities of the cucumber to the urinary tract.

Cilantro Smoothie

> 2 cups of cilantro (This is the leafy part of the coriander plant and **cooling.**)
> 1 cup of kale
> 1 cup of carrot
> 0.5 teaspoon of cumin
> Blenderize to pleasing consistency.
> Add water as needed.

The Nature of Recipes

There is a natural tendency to look for recipes that will help you with your change in lifestyle. However, I believe that lifestyle change is hard enough without trying to start looking for different ingredients and perhaps an entirely new way of cooking dishes. Although new recipes can be fun to explore, making new dishes may interfere with your primary focus, which is to eliminate the foods that harm you.

If you make this nutritional lifestyle transition too hard, after a while the mind will begin to complain that the change is too difficult. Later you may find yourself tossing all the recipes into the garbage and the nutritional information with them. So the best advice on how to use this nutritional information is to work it into your own current lifestyle of eating.

Be easy with this process and realize that this transition of removing foods in the No column requires time. Instead of wishing you could have such and such a food in the No column, begin looking for foods in the Moderation or Yes columns that can serve as substitutes. You should give yourself at least six weeks to begin to ease into this new way of choosing foods, but fortunately as you do this work you will begin to feel better, and that will allow you to gain more trust in the process.

Developing Nutritional Skill

From an energy perspective, the most important thing in nutrition is to become aware. As I have said, the food lists are not rules but guidelines to serve as tools for witnessing awareness. Your natural state is to be aware, but to be consciously aware means that you deliberately make choices and determine what the consequences are in the mindbody.

You are taken out by the activity of the mind through distraction and confusion. If you want to hone your awareness, it is like anything else. You have to train yourself to be consciously aware, just as athletes train for their respective sports. So if you want to be healthy with respect to nutrition, you can train yourself to become aware of nutrition.

Would you not think it strange that Tiger Woods would never practice but just show up for tournament play? It is antithetical to human existence that you would not practice the skills you want to have in your life. And health and nutrition are skills.

It is something that you work at, not something that you hope for. And health requires that you become aware and conscious. You will never attain evolving states of health without awareness and consciousness.

But measurement can become a distraction in the whole process of becoming aware. For example, if you are constantly measuring calories and weight, you can lose your awareness of the skill in nutrition. Awareness requires attention and intention.

Attention energy is desire. You have the desire to heal IC or some chronic disease, so you direct attention to the process of health. The very fact you picked up this book to read about healing IC is because you have that desire.

The energy of intention is the process of applying the information obtained from reading the book. Intention requires commitment and discipline. How many of us have the desire for something in life, but when it comes down to doing the work to make it happen, we fall short?

The desire and intention energies were not strong enough to make the thing happen in the now. We all have the desire to see things happen in life, but unfortunately the intention energy is not always there. As this happens, your desire energy dwindles until you forget about it entirely. Intention energy causes you to seek information, because by doing the work over and over again with your desire energy, new information is obtained.

For example, when you first learned to drive a car, you felt uncomfortable. But as you repeated the activity, you became adept at driving the car as your body received more information each time you drove. You develop the skill set of driving due to desire and intention energy.

Health is nothing more than applying awareness and the energies of attention and intention to manifest the skill of being healthy. Awareness is key to healing and bringing about balance in physiology. Awareness requires healing and healing requires awareness because they are one and the same. It's a dance.

If the heart of nutrition is understanding that food is medicine, then the soul of nutrition is understanding awareness and witnessing. As you shall see, this lack of awareness of the effects of lifestyle and nutritional choices on the mindbody can lead to extremely poor health.

Foods and Healing

Foods can produce degenerative, inflammatory, and congestive changes in the body. These changes become manifested in the matter field diseases such as fibromyalgia, hyperacidity syndrome, gastroesophageal reflux disease (GERD), IBS, interstitial cystitis, and chronic prostatitis.

But by the same reasoning, foods and their combinations can be healing. Nutrition can be antidegenerative, anti-inflammatory, and anticongestive. This is the value of the energy science approach. But you need nutritional tools to help you on your journey. They direct your energies of attention and intention to keep you from being distracted.

The 5 Interrogatives of Nutrition

What: You can begin by carrying your nutritional formats and food incompatibility lists with you wherever you go for six weeks. It takes time to assimilate the information, so carry the lists to the grocery store and restaurant and when you get ready to prepare a meal. When you consult the lists frequently, you will become comfortable with the information rapidly, and after a while you won't need the lists any further, except for occasional referral.

Where: You can make a deal with yourself that you sit whenever you choose to eat anything. This does not mean sitting in the car and eating while driving down the freeway but in a quiet setting to appreciate with all five senses the experience of the food, even if only one grape.

When: Always try to eat your biggest meal between 10 a.m. and 2 p.m. The evening meal should always be less than the noon meal.

How: Awareness not only in eating the food itself but also in the selection and preparation of the food.

Why: Emotional eating occurs even if you are aware. In bringing overeating or emotional eating to consciousness, you have a chance to have a choice. There is no choice before you are aware. If you are constantly aware of overeating, there will come a time when the overeating will be seen for what it is and insight will occur about the reason for it. Then that will be the end to overeating.

Nutritional Rituals

A ritual is an activity that draws our attention to something of importance—in this case, those that evolve our health, particularly in the morning as we begin our day.

The idea of morning rituals is to awaken the body, since the sensory experience of the body provides the key to the maintenance of balance. First, you can show appreciation for the day and then splash cold water on your face to wake up. You can awaken the GI tract by drinking room-temperature water that has set over night in a copper cup. This stimulates bowel activity and hopefully stimulates colonic activity to initiate a bowel movement.

Scraping the tongue stimulates the GI tract and clears lymphatics. Once you get the excess saliva and material off the tongue, you can then read your tongue. Getting used to the crevices and lines of the tongue helps you monitor your healing process over time. And then one day your tongue looks like that of a baby and you will have moved to a remarkable state of health that you had long ago.

Sesame oil held in the mouth for three to five minutes while doing other things in the bath helps reduce problems of periodontitis and hence heart disease. It reduces facial wrinkles because sesame oil is absorbed through the lining of the mouth. Eventually over a period the face becomes smooth. The oil helps enhance the sensory reception of the taste buds, which are the skin of the tongue. Spit the oil in the toilet, not the sink, and flush.

Monitoring Bowel Function

Monitoring how your GI tract is functioning gives you important information. It can tell you a lot about stagnation or disrupted gut elimination. The habit of observing how your body is digesting is based on fundamental observations.

The simplest assessment is observing the frequency of your stooling, the speed with which stooling occurs, the appearance of the stool, and whether it sinks or floats. Some come close to this pattern and some are very far away, but the importance here is that you recognize what is normal.

Normal Stool Pattern and Appearance

Usually early a.m. on arising
Occurs two to three hours after eating
Elimination rapid
Soft like a banana
No odor
Floats
Fragments with flushing

Due to a normal reflex, stooling occurs in the a.m. and after eating, because a message is sent from the stomach that asks the colon to empty and make room for the last ingested food. If you are fasting and not putting much into the GI tract, then of course, you would not expect much in the way of stool activity. Complete rectal evacuation should be within five seconds, and there is little residue around the anal orifice on wiping.

The stool should float and not stick to the bottom of the bowl. This represents no stagnation in the GI tract. Upon flushing the toilet, normal stool will fragment due to the proper functioning of the colon.

So this is normal function, and anything short of these observations represents constipation or diarrhea. Furthermore, symptoms of discomfort in the abdominal area before, during, or after eating are not normal.

Feeling excessively **hot** after eating, belching, rumbling in the abdominal area, acid indigestion, and foul flatus are all signs and symptoms of abnormal function that need to be addressed. Oftentimes the derangement in function is related to poor digestive fire, which I'll discuss in the next chapter.

Journaling

When you make lifestyle changes, the reports that you receive from the body are **subtle.** The matter field acts on the **gross** level and the energy field on the **subtle**

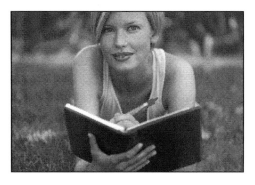

level. The nutritional changes that you make are **subtle** in nature, and it is over time that you see differences in the body.

Since matter field healing is **gross,** the expected changes occur swiftly. If you get appendicitis, matter field healing cures the imbalance expediently, and within hours you are feeling better. If an imbalance of pneumonitis occurs, then using antibiotics brings you out of your imbalance, and in a few days you are feeling better.

But energy science healing is different. The imbalances that have occurred sometimes took years and even decades to develop to their manifested state. At times healing changes occur imperceptibly **slow,** dependent on the time that it took for the imbalance to arise. It can take months or years to correct to balanced states. This leads to much confusion in assessing energy science healing when matter science tries to evaluate the use of herbs.

This **subtle** nature of healing may not be very appealing to you if you're impatient and easily frustrated, but as I have discussed, real healing can occur only over time. In the vast majority of instances, matter science healing produces a bandage and does not get to the root of the imbalance.

The use of journaling in this context can be quite helpful. When you write down observations about bowel function and then use nutritional tools to help your function, you may not see dramatic changes. But over months you will no doubt see changes for the better.

Journaling helps you look back and see that you are better than you were three months ago. For example, if you are experiencing constipation and you begin using the nutritional tools, you may over the days and weeks begin to see small improvements.

Sometimes you might see setbacks, but as you continue, you notice steady, progressive improvement. You might add an herbal bowel tonic called triphala and then use the journaling to track the improvement over time after beginning the routine use of the herb.

In this way journaling helps you see that the employed intention is bringing about the **subtle** changes in the body. Thus, journaling enhances our determination in dealing with IC. You may see in reflecting on your past urinary pattern and the flare symptoms that your IC is getting better.

Balance and Normal Energetic Eating Patterns

The energy disciplines give you guidance as how to live in harmony with Nature by ingesting those qualities that provide balance for you. The intrinsic desire of Nature is to be in balance, and so should it be yours if you are to enjoy fabulous health. You are an energy field in a greater energy field called Nature.

If you harmonize the vibrational frequencies of your mindbody patterns with those of Nature, you are that much closer to helping yourself experience extraordinary peace and harmony in your physiology. This can be your gift to the greater energy field. As you become more in balance, so does the world around you.

Chapter Summary

The matter science offers you a molecular approach to foods called diet. But there is more to nourishment than foods. When you take in the totality of nourishment, the energy science calls this nutrition.

There is much confusion around the dietary approach, leading to equivocation, mistaken food allergies, and using elimination dietary approaches. Unfortunately the latter can paint you into the corner, leading to sectoring off the food selections that are entirely appropriate.

You don't need to know the theory to get to the heart of this material about energy science nutrition. The good news is that you can go to the appendix, take the questionnaire about your mindbody makeup, and begin applying this information on a practical level right now.

The nutritional formats as outlined will solve all the mystery around what foods to eat and what not to eat. Food incompatibilities are important to observe, and developing nutritional skills can maintain your movement in the right direction toward balance.

Now let's turn our attention to the most important gift you can have for health.

Chapter 5

How Nutritional Lifestyle Behaviors Cause IC

"I have been looking for answers for IC for quite some time now. I totally have followed your advice on the Pitta diet and the aloe vera, and now I know I have control over my IC. It does not control me anymore. I am 100 percent better. I have talked to some people on the IC Network, and I feel I have been brushed off because nothing so simple could work, but it did for me. Maybe there are other therapies, but for me this really did work. I only have myself to blame for bad habits. I gave my urologist a copy of the Pitta pacifying diet and information to read. He told me he would give the diet to his other patients."

Thus far you have learned that food is viewed in a different way from which you are accustomed. Instead of viewing foods as a collection of molecules (proteins, fats, carbohydrates, vitamins, minerals), the energy science sees them as a rich distribution of qualities displayed as tastes that bring balance or imbalance for you.

And if the food choices are unbalancing, they can lead to disease, first in the GI tract and then in other parts of the body, such as IC in the urinary tract. Foods produce the flares over and over again due to the unconscious choices you make.

But the energy science model goes further with respect to just nutritional choices. It also describes how our lifestyle behavior patterns affect digestion. These choices become aides in causing further imbalance of the qualities leading to IC.

As you read in previous chapters, Pitta is the energy of transformation in the body. An aspect of Pitta is digestive fire, a vital part of the Pitta energy. Digestive fire is the transformative energy in the GI tract and body that makes use of the foods that you ingest.

Digestive fire is not only responsible for digestion, absorption, and assimilation of foods, but it also represents the ability of the body to use the energy provided to it. This is called in general terms metabolism and is a key factor in health. If you have a healthy metabolism, you have good health.

As I said earlier, nutrition is more than the evaluation of molecules. It must also take into account your ability to make use of the foods that you consume. Let's explore this concept as it relates to health.

IC and Digestive Fire (Metabolism)

The association of digestive problems with IC is well-known. IBS and GERD are commonly associated sister disease labels of the matter science. They represent problems of imbalance of qualities and of the digestive fire, which is always affected in IC. Hence energy science management of IC must address digestive fire and its health.

From a matter science view, our foods are broken down by a chemical fire, which is weak if the number of enzymes available is low. The fire in this setting is created by enzymes that break down foods so you build new cells. It is a vast, complex system of integrated and interrelated systems composed of all the enzyme and bacterial systems from the mouth to the lower rectum.

From an energy science view, digestive fire is not only an energy of transformation at the GI tract level but the hallmark of what the matter science calls metabolism. What sets apart the matter and energy sciences' understanding of metabolism is that in the former there is no association with the body's metabolism and digestion of foods.

But the energy science says that if the GI tract's central digestive fire is healthy, then the rest of the body's metabolism is healthy as well. **Wow, that's saying a mouthful!** Pause for a moment to take in what that means.

If the GI tract digestion is healthy, then all the peripheral systems, such as the thyroid and other endocrine systems, are healthy (if unhealthy, adrenal stress syndrome). If the central digestive fire is healthy, then all the remaining tissues in the body are healthy. Conversely, if the central fire is weak, so will the bodily tissues be weak.

But it goes even further. If the central digestive fire is weak, then so is our immunity. Autoimmune disease then is actually an expression of poor digestive fire. So you can see the vital importance that digestive fire holds for your own health.

The importance of digestive fire is tantamount to healing IC. Yes, it's important to correct the imbalances of qualities through the foods you take in, but equally important is to address digestive fire issues. First is the assessment of the health of digestive fire and second is how to improve it if it is not up to par.

Mary's Story
*In the throes of a flare, Mary notices that her digestion seems to go awry. There's definitely more burping after a meal, and she finds that her occasional acid indigestion is more pronounced, such that she has to use Tums or Rolaids. Sometimes the symptoms may even predate the beginning of her flare. She finds that she has no appetite but feels as if she should eat anyway. During the time of flare, she feels **heavy** and **dull,** as if there is a weight on her abdomen.*

Assessment: Appetite and the Tongue

"How's your appetite?" With this simple but elegant question, I am asking you how your metabolism is functioning today. But specifically I am also asking how you will be digesting today.

When appetite is robust, you are ready for the experience of food, and it is most normal to have that experience around noontime as I discussed in the last chapter. You know when your body needs nutrition by your best ally for health, your appetite.

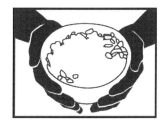

You can gauge how much is needed by using two handfuls to represent two-thirds of the stomach capacity. You can obtain a visual of this by putting a rice bowl in your cupped two hands and seeing how much this would look like in a bowl. You then can use the bowl as a gauge as to the size of your serving amount.

A second way to assess digestive fire function is to look at your tongue. The tongue's surface indicates the health of the entire body, particularly the health of the GI tract. If it is coated with a black, brown, or whitish film after scraping, it indicates that the digestive fire is not up to par. This also suggests stagnant energy in the GI tract and usually in the rest of the body as well.

I'll discuss this later on in the chapter.

The Magic Forest

For a minute I'd like to take you to a very special lush green forest. Within this forest are trees of different types, some strong, some looking young, and others mature and hearty. If the forest has brown areas and trees dying off, then the forest is deteriorating.

The digestive system can be likened to this forest, with each tree representing an enzyme or bacterial system in the long, transformative channel called the GI tract. So, for example, a tree could represent the enzyme system that breaks down lactose, and another collection of enzymes would digest gluten. But this forest is magic because it's on fire but never burns down, constantly being replenished as the fire rages.

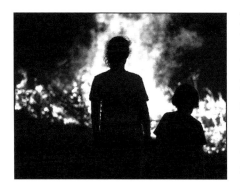

Now, a forest is a community. Each tree survives because of the community of the forest. So the trees take care of one another, and the same is true for our GI tract. The enzyme and bacterial systems are interdependent and support each other.

Because of this community aspect of your forest, it would make sense that you should nourish the entire forest, not just individual, selected trees. Feeding and watering the entire forest mirrors what you and I should do for our own GI tracts. And the energy science can help show us how to do that.

Metabolic Lifestyle Behaviors That Lessen the Digestive Fire

Since digestive fire plays such a central role for health, this list of behaviors is key to not only healing your chronic disease of IC but also to having amazing, lasting health. And even if there is a bump in the road with respect to your health, having a strong digestion will go a long way toward recovery.

Putting Out the Forest Fire

Consuming foods in the No column
Consuming incompatible foods
Consuming leftover food (>48 hours old)
Consuming raw food consistently
Consuming icy-cold drinks, cold or dry food
Consistent consumption of heavy, oily foods
Overeating: More than two handfuls of food at a meal
Snacking between meals
Excessive water intake (see Chapter 7)
Smoking and substance abuse
Emotional factors: anxiety, fear, grief, sadness, anger
Suppression of normal urges such as appetite

Assessment: Signs and Symptoms of a Healthy Digestive Fire

The signs of a good digestive fire are **subtle** compared with **gross,** obvious disease, and this would be consistent with what you know in comparing the body's energy and matter field. The below table demonstrates this.

Signs and Symptoms of Healthy Digestive Fire

Normal appetite and thirst without cravings
Subjective feeling of lightness after eating
Belching without flavors or previous eaten food
Clean tongue
Fragrant breath
Good taste perception
Proper GI tract elimination (no diarrhea or constipation)
Steady weight
Normal urination

Good visual perception

Normal temperature

Healthy color luster and glowing complexion

Well-nourished tissues

Normal immunity

Vigor, vitality, strength, and stamina

Healthy glow and luster

Mental clarity and wholeness

Sound sleep

Alertness

Discrimination intelligence

Direction, determination, and appropriate goals

Courage and confidence

Joy, cheerfulness, and contentment

Affection and enthusiasm

Patience

Enhanced longevity, maintenance of life span

Assessment: Signs and Symptoms of a Poor Digestive Fire

But what happens if the magic of your forest fire is laboring and trees are burning down slowly? The symptoms of poor digestion, which are equally **subtle,** begin to appear.

Signs and Symptoms of Poor Digestive Fire

Acute (Short-term) Signs and Symptoms

Poor appetite

Coated tongue

Nausea

Weakness and fatigue

Foul gas or flatus; bad smelling feces

Abdominal pain

Chronic (Long-term) Signs and Symptoms

> Bad breath
> Tissue emaciation
> Malabsorption
> Emotional eating
> Food cravings
> Food allergies
> Insomnia
> Poor visual perception
> Poor circulation
> Abnormal color and complexion
> Lack of luster
> Fear
> Grief, sadness, depression
> Confusion
> Apathy, repulsion
> Indecisiveness and lack of discrimination
> Lack of intelligence
> Impatience
> Shortened life span
> Improper direction and inappropriate goals

Digestive Fire and Food Allergies(Gluten and Lactose Intolerances)

No doubt food allergies to nuts or other foods are real. And the responses can be significant as a life threatening anaphylactic reaction can be elicited if taken internally.

But because the medical and general community doesn't understand the concept of agni or digestive fire, there is presently a clear tendency to blame foods for the symptoms of poor digestion. Certain foods we digest have very large molecules such as gluten(specifically wheat products), lactose(in all forms of dairy), and soy. If your digestive fire is weak and/or the food is improperly taken(cold milk, iced lattes) then digestive symptoms will occur but it is not the foods. IT'S YOUR DIGESTIVE STRENGTH!

For example, if you ingest gluten in the form of wheat products and then have nausea, fatigue, and foul smelling flatus 2 to 6 hours after eating there may be the conclusion that there is a gluten intolerance. Moreover when this is tested by an elimination

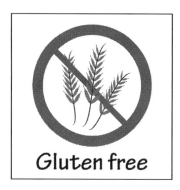

Gluten free

diet approach the after meal symptoms get better or resolve. Further the IC symptoms may get better.

When incompatible food combinations or poor digestion occurs stagnant energy or ama in the molecular form is produced as a byproduct of the digestive process. This ama over time produces a toxic sludge in the GI tract that interferes with digestion, absorption, and elimination. Even worse this ama is carried to the peripheral tissues to participate in disease processes.

Now you can see now how important digestive fire is and how if it is strong will enhance the longevity of your life and allow you to burn away "food intake mistakes." And if it is weak will lead to a toxic load in your gut. Getting rid of toxic load is part of any healing process, even with IC and its sister disease states.

This toxic load is acidic. Sound familiar? Now you understand that if you don't take care of the GI toxic load you will never clear your IC and associated conditions. And if you stop gluten you reduce toxic load and your IC flares get better.

But guess what? Your health from an energy science point of view is still highly compromised. You have dealt with the tip of the iceberg but unfortunately you remain toxic (detoxification is covered in the next chapter).

The energy science provides specific ways as to how to identify toxicity and how to begin eradicating it from the gut and body but this is beyond the scope of this text. In future books in this series this will be addressed.

Role of Spices in Enhancing Digestion

Spices are energy messages to the GI tract that stoke digestive fire. They are vitally important to our health, but unfortunately their importance is not understood. Therefore, they are not used to their full potential by the average person seeking health. There are **cooling** spices that don't provoke Pitta and heating spices that are. I'll talk about these in the next chapter.

Following the nutritional formats will give you guidance about the spices that can be used without provoking flares. If there is already too much of the **hot** quality noted by your IC, then adding a lot of **hot** spices like garlic, oregano, sage, rosemary, and thyme will provoke you into producing more flares.

Cooling spices are best for IC. These include the mints, fresh ginger (not dry), fresh basil, cumin, coriander, fennel, turmeric, saffron, and vanilla. Those that can be used in moderation include cardamom, cinnamon, dill, parsley, and savory.

In the appendix there is a section on the creation of a churan (collection of spices) that can not only stoke the fire but also bring balance to the GI tract and the body. Using a churan regularly with cooking is health promoting and helps maintain balance. This is because all six tastes are presented with this mixture.

Energy Stagnation in the Mindbody

Vata is the movement of energy in the mindbody. When it becomes excessive it moves out of the GI tract and most often carries Pitta and Kapha with it. When it stays in the tissues, it produces symptoms like cracking and popping of the joints (air in the joints leading to the **dry** and **rough** qualities), ringing in the ears, or scattered excessive movement of thought that usually results in high anxiety levels.

Causes of Energy Stagnation

> Poor digestive fire
> Accumulated wastes (urine, stool, sweat)
> Imbalanced energy patterns
> Mind interference to nutrition

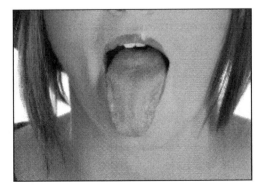

Stagnation of this energy in the body will show up on the tongue. It appears to the casual observer as a white, brownish, or blackish discoloration. The taste buds of the tongue have a very small lymph channel that loops through it, and if the channel is plugged it shows this discoloration, dependent on the energy pattern most affected.

But this Vata energy can become covered or layered over by Pitta, Kapha, or both. If Pitta is present (yellow/brown tongue change), inflammation is the result; if Kapha is present (white tongue change), lack of mobility, stiffness, or inertia of the body part or the body itself results. If Vata carries Pitta to the urinary tract, there is frequency and burning on urination. Sound familiar?

But what happens if Vata carries Kapha to the muscle and ligament layer? Then there can be stiffness and inertia of the muscles and ligaments. And as the Kapha qualities are released from the muscle with stretching and yoga, you may find that popping and cracking of the joints begins to occur due to Vata becoming uncovered.

Signs and Symptoms of Energetic Stagnation

> Fatigue
> Heaviness
> Indigestion
> Perverted taste
> Abnormal cravings
> Poor appetite
> Sexual debility
> Mental confusion
> Feeling of uncleanliness

In all of the above examples, energy becomes stagnant due to the fixation of Vata, Pitta, and/or Kapha in the tissues. When you do oleation and massage to the tissues, this stagnant energy starts flowing. The resultant qualities or sensations of **light, cold, mobile, subtle,** and **clear** (sensed as a tingling and **light**ness in the area involved) are felt. People who practice yoga can relate to this experience in receiving the body's response to a posture. This becomes apparent because Vata is becoming **mobile** and the stagnation of energy is being resolved.

Mary's Story

After hearing that the tongue can show toxicity, Mary begins examining her tongue and notices a whitish film. She tries brushing it away with her toothbrush, but it stays. It's like a stain from

*eating too much yogurt. After a week or so, she gives up and
leaves it alone.*

Cravings

Cravings can be normal because the mind wants to restore balance. If Pitta is excessively **hot**, then the craving would be appropriate for **cold** things. But when cravings are pathologic, then Pitta would be looking for **hot,** spicy foods even though it already has too much **hot** quality. This kind of pathologic craving is a result of energetic stagnation. The nervous system has loss of clarity, and as a result your mind wants something that the body doesn't need.

The movement of Vata energy becomes stuck and locked in areas, leading to the perverted or distorted food cravings that are not balancing or sound emotional choices. Interestingly, when Vata is stuck there is craving for **dry, rough** foods, such as salads and chips, as well as activities that require quick strong movement, such as jogging. Kapha develops cravings for **heavy, cold**, **smooth,** and **oily** foods. The antidote for all of these cravings is to use the opposite of what you are looking for.

As you clear the nervous system stagnation and restore the free flow of energy through the tissues, the cravings gradually dissipate. In the end, as more balance is achieved, the abnormal cravings gradually go away and are replaced by appropriate physiologic cravings. If they return, it will be transient and the antidote will be noticeably pleasing.

Role of Juicing and Fasting

Another way of thinking of digestive fire is as a campfire that you have stood around on a **cold** evening seeking warmth. If the fire is **hot** and sending out warmth and moisture, it's nourishing to you. But if you throw some wet (**slimy, liquid, dense**) logs on it, the fire quickly goes down.

When you don't ask the digestive fire to be used, your campfire continues to burn until all the wood has been burned up and the result is **hot** coals. These coals represent the remaining wood that will continue to be reduced to ash.

Juicing is a way of getting nutrients to the body without the body's need to expend a lot of energy to digest, absorb, and assimilate the food. In essence, juicing gives the

GI tract some rest and enables it to rejuvenate itself, allowing the digestive fire to get **hotter**.

Fasting is an extension of juicing. Prolonged fasts, such as for three or seven days, using fruit juices appropriate for your energy makeup can be a way of rejuvenating digestion. Without putting any more logs on the fire, the yet-undigested debris, like the **hot** coals, gets taken care of by the digestive fire.

Support of the body during a fast can take many different forms, such as water-, fruit-, and milk-only fasts. The key is who is doing the fast. Vata should infrequently fast (once every year and only during the summer), whereas Kapha can do a daily fast every month. Pitta would be somewhere in between.

The ways to reduce the digestive fire are like putting wet logs on the campfire. It is no longer able to burn the fuel that it's given. By overeating, too much wood is placed on the fire, and this as well can affect the digestion.

Ways to Enhance Digestive Fire

Follow nutritional format for body's energy pattern
Avoid incompatible food combinations
Avoid those lifestyle habits that put out the forest fire
Juice fasting
Use of ghee (see appendix)
Use of spices

Macrobiotics and Ayurveda

Hippocrates, said to be one of the fathers of current Western medicine, was the first to write about macrobiotics, describing people who were healthy and long lived (macro = long and bios = life).

A German physician, Hufeland, in the late 1700s first articulated the tradition of current macrobiotics with the basic belief that a staple of grains and local veggies was a way to live a long, healthy life. Today it also suggests nonprocessed foods. Most of the contemporary macrobiotic writings come from Japan, where balance of the yin and yang is considered vital to health, similar to the concept discussed in preceding chapters.

Currently there is very little difference between what is practiced in macrobiotics and what Ayurveda recommends. Ayurveda does allow the use of meat, while the protein in a macrobiotic program would come from a vegetarian source. As in the energy science view, there are seasonal variations that the macrobiotic discipline supports.

There are many validating reports of the success of the macrobiotic diet to help people overcome significant health challenges, such as cancer. These validations support the use of the energy science approach to healing.

Raw Foods

A lot is written about raw foods and its health benefits. The view is that the primary value in raw food is that the enzymes present in the foods are diminished or destroyed by heating. Another benefit of the raw food diet is that by not cooking the food, you keep all its beneficial qualities.

The problem with the approach is that those protein enzymes are broken down in the stomach, rendering them ineffective for digestion. Releasing the valuable nutrients from uncooked foods requires much more energy to be expended, so the net benefit is depletion of your own energy for digestion.

Ayurveda recommends cooking your food to use the heat to break down its fibrous structure and to "predigest" it so it's easier for the body to get the nutrients from the food. This is why the energy science suggests that milk should not be taken cold or used with meals, since milk is such a hard food to digest that the body needs heat and attention to do a good job digesting it.

Role of Ghee

Ghee is defined as a clarified butter, but it is much more than that. Ghee is the **oily** essence of milk. You usually don't think of milk as **oily,** but that is one of the qualities that make it a complete food (mother's milk can sustain a baby's needs in early infancy). Because of this, ghee makes an incredible cooking oil with a very high melting point.

From an energy science view, ghee stokes digestive fire because the qualities of ghee closely mimic those of digestive fire itself. Hence ghee helps support weak digestive fires in moderation. Further, ghee is a prime food to oleate the internal world of the body.

Just as the skin becomes **dry** and **rough,** so can your internal environment. Ghee penetrates the tissues twenty-four hours after ingestion, making it a great substance to oleate the internal world. This also makes it a good vehicle to carry herbs to the deeper tissues quickly. You can learn how to prepare ghee in the appendix.

Overcoming Nutritional Mistakes

But let's face it—you and I will succumb to habits, and lifestyle choices will not always be the best. At social gatherings, celebrations, or just in daily life, you may consume too much alcohol, overeat, or take in foods that provoke your energy body. So what to do?

How can we escape through life doing everything wrong energetically and still live to a reasonably ripe old age? From an energy perspective, the answer lies in this precious gift, digestive fire. It is said that the digestive fire is a key ingredient to longevity.

Athletes, when actively working out, have very strong digestive fires and clean tongues due to their strong digestion, even though they are at times eating nutrition not correct for their energy makeup.

So in the end, a healthy digestive fire, if strong and robust, will burn off our nutritional choices if they are imbalancing (chocolate, coffee) mistakes much like the robust campfire will burn down a **cold, slimy, liquid,** and **dense** wet log if placed on the fire. For Kapha, the consumption of dairy will lower the digestive fire transiently if the fire is rich, but doing this on a regular basis will lead to chronic loss of health and in the long term the health problems of obesity (**heavy, dense, soft, oily**), lethargy (**static**), and mental **dull**ness.

Chapter Summary

The energy science calls metabolism or transformation the digestive fire. You can assess your digestive fire by the symptoms you have when eating two handfuls at each meal and monitoring the surface coating of the tongue. There are lifestyle habits that can reduce your digestion and a healthy metabolic state.

Eating when there is a poor strength of digestion will bring obvious symptoms. When the system becomes debilitated, symptoms and signs of energy stagnation occur. Cravings of all kinds happen when stagnation occurs. A number of lifestyle behaviors can remedy poor digestion.

Next I'll discuss more specific treatments to manage IC.

Chapter 6

Herbs for Inflammation and IC

"I just started Ayurvedic treatment through a doctor in London about a month ago. I have severe IC and have not found any relief from the many meds and treatments I have tried. I have had severe IC for over five years, and nothing gave me significant relief until now. I cannot believe the difference. I can walk around, drive, and eat more than just a handful of foods. My life is so much better that I am thrilled. This is the first hope I have had in a long time. I am so grateful. So to anyone out there who is in pain and tried all the usual treatment to no avail, you may want to look into an Ayurvedic practitioner. It is certainly working for me."

From **IC Network** *thread, April 2008*

Thus far the Ayurvedic nutrition was outlined as a guide to improve balance and control IC symptoms. The energy science concept of digestive fire was explained, as was how metabolic lifestyle behaviors around the eating process can help improve digestion. Both of these health-enhancing broad categories of the energy science discipline are foundational to heal IC and its chronic sister diseases.

From an energy science view, not treating foods as medicine and not using metabolic lifestyle changes as methods for healing chronic diseases is problematic. Both are benign and innocuous suggestions in disease management, yet due to the current healing model, it cannot be understood how such therapies might work.

So pharmaceuticals and herbs should take a backseat to nutrition and lifestyle. Unfortunately, they have become the mainstays of therapy, which contradicts the philosophy of the energy science of Ayurveda. There is an energy science axiom that states, "If you have a strong digestion, you won't need any herbs. And if you have a weak digestion, then all the herbs in the world won't help you."

You live in a society that tells you that the answer to health is a pill. If you're sick, take a pill. And that panacea mind-set has spilled over into herbal therapy as well. Now it has become, "If you're struggling with a health problem, take a(n)…(insert herb, supplement, or pharmaceutical)."

So with that caveat, you and I should explore the world of herbs for use in IC. Used in the correct clinical setting, they can be therapeutic and adjunctive in the healing process. For example, while you are employing nutritional and metabolic lifestyle work, using aloe vera gel can cause a quick reduction in symptoms, as I talked about in an earlier chapter.

But first let's get some contemporary background on an energy science understanding of how herbs exert their physiologic effect.

Herbs and Gene Expression

Herbs energetically have their effect on you just like the environmental (foods, weather, etc.) qualities you choose. If someone chooses to eat **hot** chilies and he is already a **hot,** angry person, he will be violent by action. And his mind will be critical, judgmental, impatient, and irritable. So does it seem that the mind and your choices dictate your actions?

Since the matter science has a purely molecular approach to the body, it's not possible to have a discussion about such relationships of foods and mental behaviors simply because of the model used. Studies have linked diet to mental disorders. But the question is, "How does diet cause the mental illness from a molecular viewpoint?"

The matter science research supports the well-known concept of genetic plasticity in health and disease states. In the *Proceedings of the National Academy of Sciences,* June 2008, Ornish and Venter, et al., showed that nutrition and lifestyle modifications affected DNA expression in men with prostate cancer. Five hundred genes associated with repression of inflammation were found to turn on after three months through a process called methylation.

It is no longer tenable to hold the belief that our genes determine our fate. Ninety-five percent of our genes are influenced by lifestyle choices, which will influence your DNA's expression. But the question of mechanism remains, "How do lifestyle behavioral changes affect DNA?"

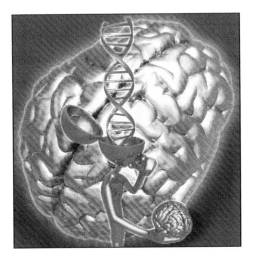

The mindbody is both an energy field and matter field—that is, both molecule and wave simultaneously. Molecules are expressions of energy, and energy can be expressed as molecules. But if the mind is an energy field, where is it molecularly?

DNA as energy is the **subtle**st molecular expression of mind. Being predominantly an energy field, mind defies a matter science molecular definition. Have you ever tried wetting a thought in the shower? Physically, it's not possible.

From the energy science model, mind or DNA is constantly eavesdropping on everything that's going on from the external (e.g., weather) and internal (foods) environment, and it's influenced by qualities that include herbs. Literally these qualities cause shape-shifting of your DNA, altering its gene expression due to this eavesdropping.

Qualities affecting gene expressions are responsible for your lifestyle behavior patterns that create either balance (health) or imbalance (chronic disease like IC). When you change your DNA, you change your mind, and when that happens you change the way you heal and choose. Shape-shifting DNA affects how you think and what choices you make in the future.

You make changes in your life because of DNA spurring you on. The reason the DNA directs that change is not happenstance. It occurs because of different choices due to influential qualities that affect its expression.

That is to say, guided to make different balancing lifestyle choices, you change the way you act and heal. But notice that it's the qualities from foods among other qualitative influences that cause your actions to be different. So if you change the qualities by making balancing choices, you act more balanced and healthy automatically. And this is all mediated through your shape-shifting DNA.

As the saying goes, "It's a no brainer (literally)."

So How Do Herbs Work?

Herbs are concentrated foods, and like foods they have their impact by the qualities they give you. The qualities are the energetic messengers delivering messages to your DNA. For example, the herb aloe vera imparts the **cold** quality to counter the **hot** quality of IC and its inflammatory sister diseases.

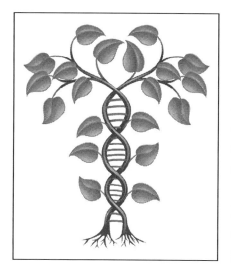

This is, of course, an oversimplification, but it gives you an idea of how qualities energetically interact with DNA and as a result have far-ranging physiologic effects. The rule is that herbs have specific targeted organ responses, but they are also used for their medicinal effects in other areas of the mindbody that do not seem to have any relationship at all to the targeted effect.

For example, turmeric—a widely used herb in cooking as well in herbal formulae—works at targeted sites such as the GI tract, circulatory, and respiratory systems. But because of its diverse DNA effects, it can be effective as an anti-inflammatory in treating IC and its sister inflammatory diseases.

Five Ways to Influence Your DNA through Energy Science Work

1. All of Nature has mind and so herbs carry mind and alter DNA expression. This is the new paradigm. Unlike molecular crystalline pharmaceuticals, herbs have specific qualities to influence DNA and in the long term have the ability to shape lifestyle behaviors.

2. As you have heard, nutrition and its qualities are heard by your DNA, and over time they have the capability to alter lifestyle behavior patterns.

3. Physical exercise, as you will learn in chapter 7, can change DNA expression.

4. Oil massage changes DNA expression, leading to health (see chapter 7).

5. Marma point therapy is identical to acupuncture and done consistently will direct differences in DNA expression (see chapter 7). The bladder marma point is effectively used when using castor oil packs (see later discussion).

Now let's look specifically at herbs and how they influence DNA.

Herbs and Their Classification

The energy science of Ayurveda states that everything that you see is capable of being medicine, given the appropriate circumstances. Whether it's a spice you recognize, such as fresh basil in the kitchen; a pharmaceutical, such as amitryptiline, which is commonly prescribed for IC symptoms; or aloe vera that you've used for sunburns, all are definable as medicines. Nonprescription herbs are commonly foreign to you but are valuable adjuncts to nutritional and behavioral lifestyle work.

The world of herbs is a complex topic, but for your purposes it can be broken down into three broad categories. The first are spices commonly used in cooking. This may be surprising to you, but they are extremely important from an energy science view, as they enhance digestive fire in all its various aspects of function.

The second category is composed of therapeutic herbs that solve very specific problems, such as IC. Taken alone they are not as effective, but done with nutritional and metabolic lifestyle work they can be highly efficacious. For example, aloe vera when combined with a Pitta-reducing nutritional format can have an almost immediate (one to two weeks) impact on flares.

The third category is a special group of herbs that are rejuvenative. These herbs restore youthful vigor and vitality. Call this revival the fountain of youth if you will, but as I just explained, little herbal rejuvenation can be noted unless you are willing to do the foundational work. The use of this type of herbal therapy is described below.

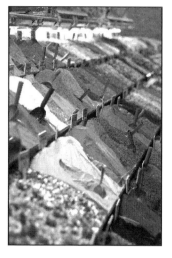

Spices as Herbs

In general, spices add extra medicine to the medicinal food so you can digest better. In the discussion of digestive fire earlier, you saw the primary importance of the GI tract in disease and how being able to digest food well and completely leads to good health. Hence the kitchen spice drawer becomes a medicine cabinet.

Interestingly, even though spices as herbs can enhance digestive fire, there is a class of spices that have a **cooling** effect while others have a **heating** effect. As a group they can balance the **hot** that is abnormally present in the GI tract. This has great relevance for IC patients who have the excess **hot** quality already.

Cooling Digestants Good for IC

Fresh basil	Fresh ginger	Tumeric
Cardamom*	Coriander	Cumin
Dill	Fennel	Mint
Rosewater	Saffron	Vanilla

*Use in moderation.

Using heating spices can only make things worse for IC. This is a good time to say that the herbal effects typically don't act like what you have experienced with pharmaceuticals. The physiologic effects take time to manifest and are **soft** and **subtle** in their expression.

Heating Digestants

Ajwan	Cloves	Nutmeg
Thyme	Allspice	Dry ginger
Oregano	Almond extract	Dry basil
Parsley	Anise	Fenugreek
Poppy seeds	Asafetida (hing)	Garlic
Rosemary	Bay	Horseradish
Sage	Black pepper	Mace
Salt	Cayenne	Marjoram
Savory	Cinnamon	Mustard
	Tarragon	

But spices are also herbs, concentrated foods that have specific medicinal effects for you. Wherever there is an imbalance, spices as herbs can have a pronounced effect, leading over time to greater levels of balance. This is in part related to the fact that the use of spices with foods enhances the GI tract's digestive fire, which increases the metabolic transformative energy throughout the entire mindbody, all the way to the cellular level.

The Use of Churans

A churan is a group of spices mixed together to give a specific taste or medicinal effect. Garam masala is an example of the former, where a spicy warming to the food is imparted. In the latter medicinal category, a churan can give all six tastes at each meal and at the same time help with digestion.

This is a good place to say that as important as the use of appropriate foods in the management of IC is, it's equally important to treat the digestive imbalances that have led to the IC in the first place. The use of the churan is a way to begin that kind of GI tract healing. To not address the GI tract and its return to health and focus only on the symptoms is to address only half the problem.

The specific churans for PV and PK are listed in the appendix along with the proportions of each spice in the mixture. When you use this mixture on a regular basis it will enhance your digestion over time, which means years not weeks or days. Believing you will completely resolve IC within a matter of weeks with these tools is actually a form of denial.

Herbs as Powder or Tablets

The energy science of Ayurveda feels that taste is everything. Why? Because tastes of foods and herbs carry the qualities that create balance in the mindbody. And these qualities are delivered to the mindbody's energy field instantaneously, whether noted or not when they enter your field of awareness.

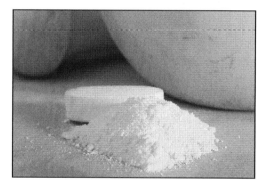

The moment that herbs touch the tongue they are delivering quality messengers to your DNA. Shifts begin to occur simply when the tastes of the herbs taken in are noted. Where does that leave tablets and capsules?

Since tablets and capsules bypass this significant aspect of taste, they cannot impact the physiology as well. Hence if given the choice between a tablet of triphala and powdered triphala, I'd suggest doing the latter. You can get over the taste and begin to experience and look forward to its nuances after a while.

And these nuances of taste are **subtle** because they come as feedback to us as to what direction our health is headed. For example, noting that the sweet taste craving is no longer dominating your life is of value. Even more **subtle,** however, is the nuance that triphala tastes sweet. Then it's time to stop triphala.

There are reputable businesses that offer excellent herbal products at reasonable prices and that are steeped in the energy science tradition. The <u>Ayurvedic Institute</u> and <u>Banyan Botanicals</u> are such companies that I would trust, and they offer powdered herbs for purchase.

Anti-inflammatory Herbs That Aid in Healing IC

Many herbs can be adjunctive in healing IC, but they should be used in the context of who is the person using them. By now you know that each of us is a unique expression of VPK, and this can change the use of an herb suggested. And even though IC is the common disease label being treated, the person has unique imbalances that may dictate the use of one herb over another.

Having said that, there is a unique aspect to the prescribing of herbs that are commonly used in IC. I have heard people talk about allergy to certain herbs, and while I don't discount those experiences, I would say that allergies are very uncommon. Oftentimes the "allergy" is a result of other products being taken and not the herb in question, but this must be sorted out an individual basis. As I wrote earlier, allergy is most often related to poor digestive fire.

Aloe vera (kumari, Aloe barbadensis)

This herb is an excellent choice for inflammatory conditions of all kinds and can be used by all mixes of VPK. As mentioned earlier, certain herbs can be rejuvenative, and aloe is one of them. This enhances its tonifying quality to tissues. It specifically balances the **hot** quality due to its **cold** quality.

Aloe can be used with pomegranate juice, which augments its anti-inflammatory characteristic. The skin of the aloe plant should not be ingested so the whole fillet preparation is best. The skin contains materials that lead to diarrhea. Dosing is one to two tablespoon three times per day.

Aloe vera is best used as a gel due to its slow release in the GI tract such that it lavages the gut mucosa in the upper intestinal tract (i.e., the stomach and small intestine). The natural thickener carrageenan is used to make it thicker, hence making it a gel. At times there has been consumer concern that carrageenan could be carcinogenic or that it would irritate IC. Although it is a saltwater plant, which energetically would aggravate IC, in the amounts that it is used it is likely safe.

Ginger (ardrakam, Zingiber officinale) Called the universal medicine, ginger as an herb can be used dry or fresh. When used dry it has a **hot** quality and therefore would not be beneficial in IC. Since it promotes digestive fire, it is a digestant in cooking. In its fresh form, it is medicinal to GI tract function.

Ginger can be used as an appetite (indicator of digestive fire) stimulant by using a quarter-inch disc of sliced ginger soaked in lime juice with a pinch of rock or sea salt. Again, given the clinical situations, there are many different combinations with other herbs in which ginger can be used.

Turmeric (Curcuma longa, Haridra) This rhizome that is similar to ginger in physical appearance imparts yellow color to food. It is an incredible spice for inflammation, particularly for skin conditions. The spice is very safe, and you can use literally grams of it at one time without deleterious side effects.

As an herb it promotes digestive fire without overheating the system, which is a particularly valuable property in IC patients. Turmeric helps in the digestion of protein and strengthens and is balancing to all metabolic functions. It helps stretch the ligaments and therefore is helpful in the practice of yoga.

Triphala is a mixture of three different herbs—haritaki, amalaki, and bibhitaki—each respectively pacifying the energy patterns of Vata, Pitta, and Kapha. Each herb can bring balance to function of the energy patterns in the colon, small bowel, and stomach respectively. Each is a rejuvenative unto itself, which makes this mixture or formula highly effective and prescribed commonly.

There are many different ways to use these herbs separately or in combination based on the clinical situation. Dosing is half a teaspoon steeped in hot water thirty minutes before bed or, if preferred, just using the powder itself with room-temperature water.

Cumin, Coriander, and Fennel The use of these three herbs in the management of IC underscores how cooking spices are herbs, which are the medicinal extension of foods themselves. All three of these herbs are medicinal to the urinary tract, and because they are **cooling** digestants, they provide the **cold** quality to the **hot** urinary tract of IC patients.

Each seed is placed in equal amounts in a Ziploc bag, and from that one tablespoon of the mixture is used for one cup of hot water to make a tea. A larger volume can be made and placed in a thermos to sip on all day. This is a nice way to lavage the urinary tract mucosa throughout the day.

Castor oil (Ricinus communis) This herb is interesting in that its application externally is **cooling** and when used internally it is **hot**. The energy science takes advantage of this by using external packs in the pelvic region for relief of IC symptoms. Of course, the internal effect of castor is increasing bowel motility due to the **hot** quality usually leading to diarrhea, making it an effective laxative.

This treatment doesn't contradict the experience of many who have found relief by using a heating pad to the lower abdomen. Heat does have benefit in reducing muscle spasm, which is **cold, mobile, rough, dry, heavy, dense, hard,** and **sharp/penetrating**. All these qualities would respond to the **hot** quality of the heating pad.

Why not try both? Apply heat to a castor oil pack. At this point it's good to note that the application of this pack is over the bladder energy point between the pelvic bone and belly button. Adding **cooling** aromas such as rose, jasmine, and mint is beneficial.

Chamomile (Anthemis nobilis) Like the preceding CCF mixture, chamomile as a tea is a Pitta-pacifying beverage and has been used successfully for staving off IC symptoms. It is balancing to the emotions, making it particularly effective for PV patients who are having trouble coping with the waves of flare. It has an effect of sedating nerve pain.

A little fresh ginger prepared with it makes chamomile a completely balanced beverage and counters any emetic effect it might have. Externally it can be used as a poultice for nerve pains. For most medicinal purposes, its action is mild and serves as a harmonizing adjunct.

Gokshura (Caltrops, Tribulis terrestris)

Also known in the West as caltrops, this herb targets the water or urinary tract channel and is effective in reducing inflammation but is also good at reducing the incidence of stone formation. It is this latter effect that suggests that gokshura is an important herb in facilitating glycosoaminoglycan (GAG) layer formation. Its best use is in formula, but it could be used in basti (below) due to the GAG-formation enhancement.

Purnarnava(Boerhaavia diffusa)

Translated as "that which renews us" this herb also like gokshura has affinity to the urinary channel. It strengthens the kidneys and in doing so aids in our overall health and vitality. Its action is more tonifying to the kidney than to the urinary bladder and therefore would be a second line herb in dealing with straightforward IC.

Dashamula (Compound)

The name translates as the ten (dasha) roots (mula) and is a mainstay in the treatment of Vata imbalances. It is a great example of where the energy science of Ayurveda combines multiple different herbal effects to give a compounding physiologic effect or what I have termed confluent physiologic effect. The roots are boiled together and then strained with a decoction or tea as the result.

Neem (Azadiracta indica)

A very important blood purifier and detoxifier in Ayurvedic usage and is useful in ulcerated or inflamed skin/mucous membrane disorders, such as in IC. It clears away excess tissue. It should be used with discretion in those with severe debility and fatigue.

Guduchi (Tinosporia cordifolia)

An important rejuvenative for Pitta and nutritive herb to take during recovery periods. It is a potent detoxifier, buring ama without aggravating Pitta. It is a great tonic for the immune system . Taken with ghee it reduces Vata, with sugar reduces Pitta, and with honey it reduces Kapha.

Shatavari (Asparagus racemosus, Indian asparagus)

This is one of the more important herbs in reducing Pitta and used for women's Pitta imbalances around menstruation but in the IC condition is unique in its application, particularly around tea decoctions for bladder therapy below. It is a rejuvenative as well. It is useful in treating dry and inflamed mucous membranes. In addition to its Pitta pacifying use, it also soothes calms Vata.

Mahanaryan Massage Oil (external use)

This is a complex base oil infused with sixty different herbs, making it a balancing oil that treats inflammation in the tissues as well as other conditions. It is a mainstay in oleation marma therapy (see Chapter 7).

Herbal Bladder Instillations

From a matter science point of view, one of the main etiological theories of IC is that the GAG layer is damaged or compromised due to some unknown cause. Because of this theory, urologists have used many instillation therapies over the years to treat this defective GAG layer problem. Heparin and steroids have been used as rescue remedies for IC flares, along with other drugs as per the practitioner.

For thousands of years, the energy science of Ayurveda has used instillation therapy as a mainstay in introducing herbs to local problem areas of the body. The general medical term used is *basti,* which means bladder, describing how in the past the bladder of an animal was used as the bag holding the herbal tea that was delivered to the lining of an organ, whether it was the lower colon as in a traditional enema, to the bladder, or to the vagina. Basti can also be done to external localized areas of the body, such as the low back or to the eyes, delivering soothing herbs to these areas.

As has been stated earlier, the delivery of herbs for treatment for any condition is done in many different ways—orally, nasally, by way of the skin, and by basti. So the matter and energy science ways of dealing with IC in terms of topical delivery of medicines to the ailing surface of the bladder are one and the same.

But as I have explained, the energy science understanding of the origin of disease and why it manifests is different from the matter science's view. And how the energy imbalance is managed is scientifically different, since the energy science chooses the herbs for treatment based on the condition of the patient's imbalance. Hence the selection of the herbs to use is based on the imbalance of qualities causing the disease—in this case the **hot** and **mobile** qualities of IC.

But often the same logic that elicits the choice of herbs taken orally is used in choosing herbs for the bladder and vagina if instillations are to be done. Herbs such as aloe could be combined with dashamula, guduchi, and gokshura tea, with aloe used after the tea has cooled. This would be effective in reducing the **hot** and **mobile** qualities of Pitta and Vata.

Here the important divergence from the matter science view is that the energy science approach is selecting herbs that affect the energetic imbalance, not a molecular problem.

Preparation and Use of Herbal Targeted Instillations

As I have discussed earlier, the severe debility of IC involves probably about 30 to 40 percent of the population that develops symptoms. Decoctions, also known as teas, are prepared with the following appropriate herbs and instilled into the bladder or vagina.

Vaginally for vulvodynia: For Pitta (burning vaginal symptoms) use neem or guduchi with aloe; for Vata (episodic and/or fleeting pain) use dashamula root with aloe. Preparation below. Administer as a lavage to the vaginal lining.

 Intravesically for IC bladder symptoms: Use 1T dashamula root tea with 1T gokshura, with 1T guduchi, neem, or shatavari (based on predominant symptoms Vata or Pitta), and after cool, add 0.25 cup aloe vera gel. Choose two other herbs to use with the dashamula root to make 3 cups of decoction.

Preparation of decoction: Bring 0.5 cup distilled water/herb used (e.g., two herbs used = 2 cups) to boil; add the herbs; cook for five minutes then cool in freezer until warm. Then if using it, add the 0.25 cup aloe vera gel.

Administration: Use clean catheterization vaginally or into the bladder. May need to use 2 percent lidocaine jelly intraurethrally for passage of catheter on initial instillations.

NB: Due to small bladder capacity, secondary to increased Vata (**mobile**), a patient may be able to accept only 75–100cc at a time, which will require two or three instillations until all of the decoction is used. If this is the case, can reduce the volume of decoction until able to accept more.

Basti schedule based on responsiveness of symptoms: eight, fifteen, or thirty days.

Herbal Methods for Vaginal Pain

In Chapter 5 I talked about ghee, the **oily** essence of milk, and in the appendix is the simple method as to how to prepare ghee. This universal medicine is used in many different ways in Ayurveda, but it can be also used as a carrier to take herbs to parts of the body quickly. Think of it as a taxicab, with the herb as the passenger. Shatavari is a PV pacifying herb and also a rejuvenative, as mentioned above. It is excellent in high Pitta conditions and is itself a feminine rejuvenative.

As discussed above, basti is a general term for application of herbs and/or oils to various parts of the body to introduce herbs and their therapeutic value to a specific region of the body. You can make a tea with most any herb so that administration can be done.

This is the case in vaginal pain in vulvodynia and IC. The **hot** and **sharp** stabbing pain involved with intimacy can be helped by using an appropriate herbal tea administered with an enema bag into the vaginal canal similar to what would be done in douching.

Cooling herbs such as shatavari, bhringaraj, and brahmi can be used in combination or separately but should be done under the guidance of a trained Ayurvedic physician. The use of both of these methods is beyond the scope of a layperson at home, and the patient should be screened as to the appropriateness of the herb in an individual clinical setting.

Role of Detoxification

As I discussed in chapter five, ama is a type of sluggish Kapha energy that is carried to the tissues and channels by Vata. This energy becomes stagnant and interferes with the free flow of energy inhibiting healing and clearance of the excess qualities from the periphery. You saw how this can show up on the tongue.

The process of detoxification moves ama and excess qualities back to the GI tract where they can be eliminated. This is done by eating a simple food like kitchari which is discussed in the appendix. This type of nutrition is very healing to the GI tract, which gets some time off from digesting, and encourages along with external oleation and applied moist heat to bring this ama back to the GI tract for elimination. These simple detoxification techniques can not only improve the herbal effect below but also enhanaces their effectivenss.

More Than One Route for Herbs

In herbal therapy, using more than one route of administration of the herb is more effective than simply taking the herb orally, for example. The use of herbal oils called tailams during self-directed oil massage along with an oral formula specifically tailored for the patient's imbalances would be more effective than the oral formula alone. But the use of basti-administered herbs into the bladder would be another introductory route that would produce another conveyance for the healing herb to be introduced.

In the matter science, pharma drugs have such potent effects that usually one route suffices. Alternative routes of administration, such as with a suppository in the anal canal, is chosen because in the case of vomiting the oral route of administration is compromised. But the problem with pharma in general is that these molecular packages have lost their mind. They have been altered to the point that the drug is a physiologic signal messenger to the body to do a specific activity.

In the energy science, herbs are used to ask the mindbody to make shifts in not only bodily functions and processes but also, as I discussed earlier, to produce shifts that cause the patient to make healing choices that would not have been otherwise entertained. Having several routes of administration compounds this physiologic affect such that more progress in healing can occur.

Partial Remissions

As you may have heard, there are many different ways to reach your destination in healing IC. Some get better with diet alone. Some with acupuncture. Some get well without anything being done. Most improve with combination treatments. But unfortunately for the majority of patients with IC, symptoms linger even if remission occurs (i.e., the partial remission).

Typically, because you don't know that complete resolution of IC symptoms is possible, it's reasonable to accept partial remission. If the symptoms are not severe, you have to put up with only occasional bothersome urgency and frequency. Then life is good. Perhaps more to the point: If the urologist can do occasional fulguration of ulcers, tolerable DMSO or hydrodistention treatments, or pharmaceuticals do the trick, then why bother with other work?

The best answer to this is that the imbalance that creates the low-grade IC can show up elsewhere.

Mr. Doe was a fifty-year-old white male who underwent a radical prostatectomy for high-grade disease and had a good result. He was counseled on various tools that he could use to reduce inflammation in the urinary tract and to stop smoking. Approximately five years later he returned with large stone in the left renal pelvis and was successfully treated. Then two years later he came back with a right renal cancer. The cancer was removed but three years later he died of metastatic renal cancer.

This is a tragic story of someone who could not deal with his imbalances and eventually succumbed to them. Partial remissions are merely clearing part of the tip of the iceberg, leaving imbalancing qualities still present. These kinds of states can usher in new diseases that can become problematic.

This new view of what it means to be healthy creates a new paradigm around the concept of health not necessarily held by your current matter science system of healing. Guided by this model of healing, the majority of patients with chronic disease have the goal of reducing symptoms and making life more tolerable.

But the energy science suggests that IC as a chronic disease is a valuable learning experience to bring about a healthy state beyond the symptoms of the disease. Hence IC becomes a great teacher for us if you can stand to be in the classroom with her. It's all a choice.

Management of the Acute IC Flare

As I discussed in Chapter 3, flares will gradually become less intense as you do energy science work. But how to manage these symptom flares when they do occur? The first is to realize that you have to provide the body the chance to release the Pitta energy pattern that is provoked. This requires time but doing a maintenance program helps the body do a slow release.

A maintenance program is as follows:

Staying on the nutritional format appropriate for your energy makeup and avoiding incompatible food combinations.

Regular use of aloe vera gel even when not having symptoms.

Regular use of CCF tea.

Regular exercise (see chapter 7).

Regular meditation (see appendix).

During an acute flare, here are things that you can do to help resolve the flare quicker:

Continue doing the maintenance work.

Consider simple nutrition such as kitchari (see appendix) so as to not overtax the GI tract. Emhasizing **cool**ing foods such as coconut, fresh mango, sweet fruits is therapeutic for IC, but be sure to keep the fruits separate from other foods categories.

Trying the **cool**ing drink recipes in Chapter 4 can be helpful in giving nutrition but also helping with **cool**ing the body off during this **hot** release.

Castor oil packs over the bladder area along with **cool**ing aroma oils such as jasmine, sandalwood, peppermint, and rose attars can be effective. The addition of a heating pad can help reduce the abdominal wall spasm that can occur with a flare.

Applying pressure to marma points can be effective. In the next chapter I discuss specific points referable to the bladder under **Marma and Therapeutic Oleation**.

Getting plenty of rest during these energy draining times is very valuable and avoiding any exercise.

Try using simple breathing techniques such as shitali or shitkari that can bring about **cool**ing to the body as mentioned in chapter 7.

Consider meditation (twenty minutes in the morning and evening) if the flare symptoms are not severe to reduce the excess Vata energy. For the best results use meditation as a maintenance program so that when the flare comes you'll be ready.

Consider a **cool**ing oil massage using a Pitta and Vata pacifying oils before showering.

If you live in a **hot** climate such as Florida, Texas or the Southwest, it's important to stay out of the heat. Use sunglasses as often as possible.

Swimming can be **cool**ing for a flare but not in midday when it may be **hot** out.

Stay **cool** (anti Pitta), calm (anti Vata), trying to reduce impatience (Pitta) and irritability (Pitta) as much as possible.

Try not to judge, control, or blame others and minimize perfectionism.

If tolerated a targeted herbal bladder instillation at your urologist's office may help particularly if the flare symptoms are not severe and incapacitating.

The Good News about IC

The urinary tract, like the GI tract, is actually a long tube beginning at the glomerulus of the kidney and ending at the urethral opening. The qualities that I have discussed previously may energetically disrupt the lining of the channel. This is reminiscent of the GAG layer matter science discussions, which say that this layer becomes in some way deficient, but it is unknown why or how.

Even though the qualities affect the lining of the tube, they don't do as much damage as when they involve tissues such as the muscular layer in fibromyalgia or the nervous system as in Parkinson's disease. There are situations where the lining of the urinary tract tube can be involved at deep levels, such as in bladder cancer, but this is not the case with IC. And matter science epidemiologic studies show that there is no correlation between IC and bladder cancer.

Since IC is a superficial, qualitative problem in the urinary channel, it has a good chance of being healed based on what we know from an energy science view. This is a nice gift that the energy science has for IC patients who understand their disease in a different way. Then there can be hope.

Chronic Prostatitis

The symptoms of chronic prostatitis have to be sorted out by a urologist with an open mind. From an energy model view, there may indeed be qualitative changes occurring in the genital system, which as I just said makes the disease more difficult to treat but still not impossible. But the treatment will be different and more pro-longed, as in fibromyalgia.

The current issue of PSA (prostate specific antigen) is actually an inflammatory condition but has been used as nonspecific marker for prostate cancer. PSA is a marker for inflammation, not cancer. It measures the **hot** quality. By using an anti-inflammatory approach, PSA can be reduced.

Prostate cancer is an inflammatory disease like all cancers. And like all cancers, all three energy patterns become localized in the prostate tissue, leading to the expression of high- or low-grade disease. The conundrum facing matter science doctors today is how to treat the low-grade, apparently small-volume disease.

My bias is that in appropriate patients, an anti-inflammatory approach can heal low-grade, small-volume prostate cancer. Of course, this kind of therapy has to be monitored carefully and in a research setting. This kind of thought process born out of the energy science discipline shows the value of integration of the two healing models.

But chronic prostatitis may not involve the prostate tissue itself. The qualitative change may be involving only the lining of the urinary tract. In this case, an anti-inflammatory approach could be exactly what is needed to clear symptoms.

Benign enlargement of the prostate, which produces a Kapha congestive component, can make the urological interpretation of symptoms difficult to sort out for those experiencing lower tract irritative and obstructive symptoms. It's easy if the prostate gland is small (twenty grams or less), but as the gland gets larger, then this congestive component may play a role in symptoms.

With all the above said, changes in voiding patterns that occur in men as they progress in years are typically related to inflammatory energy changes in the urinary tract and are usually not obstructive. Unless the obstructing tissue is large in volume, inflammation explains why men often are not helped with surgery for removing "obstructive tissue." Symptoms of obstruction were actually irritative (inflammatory) in nature.

Chapter Summary

From an energy science perspective, nutrition and metabolic lifestyle behavior changes are core to healing any chronic disease, including IC.

Herbs can offer immediate relief in some situations and support the nutrition and metabolic lifestyle behaviors in the long term. But herbs, like pharmaceuticals, are not primary but secondary in management. This is a clear departure from current thinking about disease management but is tantamount to success in dealing with chronic disease.

Lastly exercise is an important adjunct in lifestyle behaviors because it stokes digestive fire. Let's look at this.

Chapter 7

Exercise the Body Quiet the Mind

*"Hope is always needed. Otherwise it's a rather
pointless journey, isn't it?"*

*"A turbulent mind is your enemy but
a quiet mind is your friend"*

Chronic disease especially when associated with pain is an energetic drain on the mindbody. The fear of the recurrence of the pain can be equally as wearing as the flare itself. With both disease and pain there is a loss of vital energy or life force and a withering of the mindbody under the torment.

As I have stated throughout in earlier chapters the relief using the energy science approach comes but it does not occur overnight. Real healing takes time. So the process of healing requires supporting the mindbody as it pulls itself out of the ditch.

The value of supporting the weakened mindbody in healing from painful chronic disease is similar to the support required in challenging cancer chemotherapy protocols. I have talked about the use of herbs that can play a supportive role in the last chapter but the energy science of Ayurveda offers many other rejuvenative techniques that support the mindbody in healing. So in this last chapter that you and I have together I want to give you some appreciation of what kinds of mindbody supporting techniques are available to you.

Exercising the Physical Body

When it comes to exercise in our culture, you are taught that benefit comes only with "pain yields gain." But if you look at the life expectancy of athletes, it's apparent that longevity is not assured due to the athletic training. From an energy science point of view, although exercise itself is important, it should be tempered by who you are energetically.

Vata-predominant people should do light exercise which do not require a lot of stamina, such as long hikes or distance running. Even though it's popular for Vata to engage in marathons, the joints cannot handle that kind of punishment long term. Such exercise as yoga, dance, and Pilates are excellent choices.

Pitta-predominant people should do moderate exercise. Due to the excess **hot** quality, swimming is a great choice. Due to the competitiveness of Pitta, there is a strong need to choose a sport activity where winning is the reward, such as racquetball, tennis, soccer, and organized sports. Actually it's better that Pitta stay out of competitive exercise and focus on the individual enjoyment of the exercise. So swimming for the pure enjoyment of being in the pool would be best.

Kapha-predominant people can and should do strenuous exercise with lots of movement. Typically you see strong Kapha people doing weight lifting because they're good at it, but Kapha needs to *move,* and doing more aerobic workouts is beneficial. Kapha joints can withstand long-distance running, and it's an excellent exercise for this energy pattern.

And by the way each energy pattern has different fluid requirements. Since you have IC, you have been told that you should drink large volumes of fluid to dilute the nasty molecules that are causing your symptoms. Most cannot do that, due to the frequency and urgency that occurs with increasing diuresis. Vatas should drink seventy ounces per day, Pittas sixty ounces, and Kaphas forty to fifty ounces. Overconsumption by Kaphas simply leads to congestion and weight problems. Again, when dealing with combination energy patterns, adjustments can be made (e.g., PV sixty-five ounces versus PK fifty ounces).

You're combinations of these energy patterns, as you'll see when you take the questionnaire. Your makeup of two energy patterns will help you sort out which combination exercise pattern is best for you. PV and PK will differ, but one thing you can be assured of as an IC patient is that leaving out the competition in your exercise routine is beneficial due to the Pitta aggravation caused by it.

The energy science also helps with what kind of exercise is best for mindbody make-up in another way. Recall that I said that the mind and body are intimately spliced, and that's why it's called a mindbody. If you want to exercise the body, you take it for a run, lift weights, or do something else physically.

But what about the mind? What do you do to exercise the mind? The energy science says that the best exercise for the mind is to do nothing. Nothing? Yes, because the healthiest mind is one that is quiet. That's a balanced mind. Not a hectic, frantic, got-to-move-mind, but a quiet, calm mind.

And when you calm the mind, you calm the body. So you need to exercise the body but find time to quiet the mind as well. It's again balance that I've been talking about since Chapter 2.

The Breath

Whatever exercise you are using, it's best done by paying attention to the breath. In the energy science tradition, breathing is the movement of awareness. So if you are exercising by paying attention to the breath, you're more aware of how the body is doing during the exercise. How does this look?

When you use the breath, you become aware of yourself watching. This is called witnessing, but in reality it is simply noticing yourself, which is a requirement for healing. You begin to develop a relationship with a part of yourself that may be unfamiliar to you. In the end, you are cultivating self-love by this process.

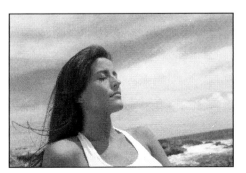

So the breath moves the body. Begin practicing watching the breath and pay attention to these details. On taking in a deep breath (inspiration), the ankles flex, the knees bend, the lower back goes forward, the torso and back extend (stretch) upward, the upper back around the shoulders goes back, the neck extends and the head goes back slightly, the arms at the elbows soften, and the hands rotate out with palms facing forward.

On letting the breath out (expiration), the ankles and knees straighten, the back and torso hold, shoulders drop and stay back, the neck flexes down, the arms straighten at the elbows, and the hands rotate back so their tops are facing forward. You can see that inspiration is very active, but that expiration seems passive. But if you watch, you will see that expiration is also very active, since it requires strength to hold the body in the extended position that inspiration produced so you don't cave in. This is a major reason for posturing of the aged that you see.

When you become a student of the breath, you will become naturally oriented in space. If proper body alignment is not maintained, poor posturing over time can occur, and no one will tell you. But if you're conscious of the breath and how it moves the body, you will be able to know when you're not in proper alignment.

So now employ this breath watching with all your activity—sitting, standing, walking, jogging, swimming, weight lifting, and best of all yoga. Yoga is a beautiful way to teach yourself how to watch your body in all kinds of different positions using the breath.

Just as the breath becomes a tool as to how to align yourself in space during all activities, unconditional love becomes the tool as to how to align yourself in relationships. When you hold no judgement (emotion with a thought), resist blaming others for your problems, criticize nothing that occurs, then you begin to find a deeper reality where under no conditions is it not possible to see yourself in all of your experiences.

For example, let's say someone is angry with you. For Pitta the natural reaction is to react and respond back with anger. But with unconditional love, under no conditions will you have nothing but love for the person, no matter how angry they get.

Core Strength and the Breath

The breath is intimately associated with the strength and appearance of the body. There is one more aspect of the body in space, but core strength also needs to be addressed. The body must be prepared to receive the breath. And people in all types of professions involving physical activity, such as professional dancers, use this concept of core strength.

Although spoken about in yoga classes during asana practice, I find that the concept—while very important—is not taught. It is rather assumed that since you're in the yoga class that you have brought that knowledge with you. And like many physical features of posture, I find you either have these intuitively developed in your physiology or you don't.

The concept of core strength is often taught through poses that enhance the core, but it is not explained much. Anatomically the core is composed of the abdominal muscle (transversus abdominus), which wraps your abdominal torso from the spine to the abdominal anterior (front) midline, as well as the iliopsoas muscle in the back along with other smaller muscle groups such as the multifidis. When you engage the core, you are contracting these muscles.

What does it feel like to engage the core? It's like tensing the abdominal wall (transversus). When you engage the core, you may feel as if the torso extends and you feel taller.

Now that you've engaged the core, the next thing to do is breathe. You've prepared the body for the breath, so now it's time to breathe. The inspired breath begins at the diaphragm at the top of the abdomen as the core holds position. Near the end of inspiration, the lower abdomen near the pubic bone comes out naturally, and at the height of inspiration the sternum is lifted as if it has three balloons attached to it and they are pulling it up. It's as though the front of the abdomen has been unzipped.

Expiration is like zipping the abdomen back up while still maintaining the core strength. Do this in two phases: from the pubic bone to the umbilicus and then from the belly button to where the breath was initiated on inspiration.

When you master breath with the core, you can move into holding the core during walking, sitting, and moving through various daily activities. Then if you're interested in yoga asana practice, paying attention to the core is another excellent way to maximize your practice and progression.

Another good way to develop core strength is through kapalabhati, a breathing exercise discussed later that is said by some to be neither heating nor **cooling**.

Breath Exercises for Calming and Cooling

There are yogic breathing techniques that yield significant physiologic benefits when practiced over time. As with all energy science therapies, they can be antidegenerative (Vata), anti-inflammatory (Pitta), and anticongestive (Kapha).

Vata: Anulom villom, Nadi shodana are both alternate nostril, the former forceful exhalation; Bhramari or Bumblebee breath. All calm the nervous system and hence reduce movement in the physiology.

Pitta: Shitali and shitkari are variations of the same breathing technique and are **cool**ing.

Kapha: Bhastrika is heating and should be avoided. Kapalabhati does not overheat and so is good to use in IC even though it's considered a Kapha-pacifying breath.

You can perform an Internet search for these terms and find YouTube videos that show demonstrations of the techniques. Another way of seeing demonstrations is going to Ayurveda.com and looking for pranayama under Books and DVD. DVDs are also available at ic-solutions.com.

Meditation

You may be aware of how IC produces not only physical fatigue but now it is no surprise that as a result you experience mental fatigue as well. This translates into loss of clarity, difficulty in decision making, loss of confidence, and anxiety. Everything becomes tentative due to this energy drain. Meditation can give you the mental rest that you need.

When you sit and watch the breath, you become meditative, according to the energy science of Ayurveda. Meditation is an excellent way to calm the disturbed Vata energy pattern, which is part of the IC problem. Since Vata disorders account for 80 percent of visits to the doctor, Vata becomes a major player in disease causation and its management in disease prevention.

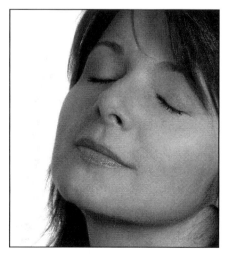

When you do this kind of breath work on a regular basis, your mind will become quiet. This is a great gift of meditation because, as I talked about earlier, it is the turbulence of the mind that produces the turbulence of the body, since they are intimately spliced. This relationship has the potential of causing disease or maintaining your disease state of IC.

It's beyond the scope of this book to go into all of the benefits of meditation, of which volumes have been written. Ongoing matter science studies are still uncovering untold physiologic benefits of the practice. The key is to do it on a regular basis. Doing it sporadically will not pay off as much as setting a regular schedule. Please see the appendix for more information about the practice.

You will come a long way by simply paying attention on a regular basis to the breath during the day with bodily movements. This is meditative in and of itself. However, lying or sitting for twenty minutes a day morning and evening is a more formal meditative practice. Vata predominant people do well with movement meditation such as yoga practice or bringing breath awareness to all daily activities such as walking, cooking, and working.

If you can't sit or lie down (before sleep or on waking) for twenty minutes, try five and then gradually increase the length of time until you are doing the full twenty minutes. Why is twenty minutes selected as a preferred time? It's been shown experientially that it takes about this long for the mind to settle into its normal, quiet state.

Mantra meditation can be added to the preceding breath-awareness-seated meditation by simply adding "so" on inhalation and "hum" on exhalation. The reason for adding the use of the mantra is to capture the busyness of the mind and give it something to chew on. Other mantras can be used as well, but these are not associated with breath awareness.

The importance in breath awareness meditation is not what happens on inhalation or exhalation but what happens in the "stops," the pauses between the two phases of breathing. In these stops is the stillness that you're looking for, the slowing down of the Vata movement of the mind. Believe it or not, this type of work has the same effect as eating foods that reduce Vata movement.

Who would think that simply quieting the mind would deal with the overactive bladder disease label?

How could this be? Taking in foods that increase the qualities of **light** and **mobile** increases movement in the physiology. When you reduce mental activity, you reduce the **mobile** quality as well. Now you can see how the mind and body are intimately related and how foods and not doing can be medicine.

How is this important for patients with IC? If you reduce the Vata energy of movement, then you can over time reduce urinary frequency and urgency. But Vata can push Pitta. So decreasing Pitta by reducing Vata can reduce the symptoms of burning in the pelvic area over time.

As I have said before, the key in energy science management is to use all the tools, not just one or two. **Confluence of healing activities** is important to make strides in healing. The cause of your IC is multifactorial, and the healing of it will occur because you use multiple approaches: nutrition, observance of incompatible food combinations, metabolic behaviors around the eating process that enhance digestive fire, use of herbs, observing appropriate rest and a day in balance, exercise, meditation, and breath awareness.

It is then that real healing of IC and its sister diseases can take place with time.

Yoga Nidra

Translated as yogic sleep, yoga nidra is a special state of rest induced by a practitioner who can guide you to a resting state that mimics but is not sleep. In this state you get a deeper state or relaxation in which the mind is receptive to desires and needs that you're interested in achieving in your life.

It is mentioned here because it is part of the yogic energy science tradition and is actually a guided meditation that can be quite useful for those who have difficulty with seated meditation. It has the physiologic benefits of a meditative practice but can also be used to access areas of the thinking process that can help program yourself for achieving tasks.

There are guided yoga nidra programs available online but the best situation is that yoga nidra sessions be built around the relief of IC rather than a generic templated yoga nidra.

Faith Trust Cycle

In energy science work it's not about believing me. It's about making the observations that by doing the work you're getting better. This enhances your trust in the discipline.

You see your faith in an energy science mode of healing is entirely in your hands and no one else's. If you see results some trust occurs and then more faith. As you go along there will more improvements and more trust with more faith. If you're being attentive and aware which is brought about by a quiet mind this will be the case.

The energy science approach to healing requires commitment on your part. This is in part brought about by a quiet, nonjudgmental, patient and noncritical mind. The mind will get in the way using doubt, indecision, and inertia to leave you without the benefits that you're seeking.

The Pitta mind when unbalanced is unduly skeptical, emotionally judgmental, impatient, and irritable. What drives this mental activity is fear. Fear of being duped, taken advantage of, and being wrong since Pitta is a perfectionist. The use of understanding yourself as an energy pattern is that it gives you an objective tool to observe yourself without condemning.

When you notice yourself becoming curious without these more damaging mental activities you know you're making progress. Basically mental turmoil induced by fear interferes with the healing process.

Yoga Practice for IC

Another way to train yourself to witness or pay attention to yourself is to do yoga posture (asana) practice. When you practiced yoga postures using the breath as talked about earlier, you can become fascinated watching the breath move body parts when you pay attention to the movements during inspiration and expiration. This is the heart of yoga and its greatest teaching.

Even though going to yoga classes can be helpful, it's best if you develop a set of postures that you can do at home. Like meditation, yoga posture practice is not very valuable to you if it's done sporadically. Setting some time each day to do posture practice is a great way to start the day.

In the next sections I'll introduce yoga poses that can be helpful in balancing VPK, and you'll be able to select those that would be appropriate. These poses are readily available online, and I have provided links for them.

<u>Tibetan Rites</u> This is a set of five postures practiced twenty-one times each in a sequence. For beginning a yoga practice, these rites are a good way to develop some flexibility and strength on top of introducing your body to stretches with which it might not be familiar. Build up to twenty-one repetitions for each rite gradually and you will begin noticing differences very soon.

Strength and flexibility are aspects of Kapha and Vata respectively, and they are intimately connected to each other. You can't have flexibility without strength and strength without flexibility. The rites as well as yoga as exercise can create both.

Yoga Postures for Vata

Since Vata is the energy pattern of movement, postures that bring balance would be those that are performed **slowly** (reduces the **mobile** quality) and ground Vata (reduces the **light** and **mobile** quality). So any posture done **slow**ly and with the breath will balance Vata, but the following will bring grounding:

<u>Sun salutation done slowly</u>

Grounding poses such as malasana, prasarita paddoanasana, utthita parsvokanasana, vriksasana, and paschimottanasana.

Yoga Postures for Pitta

Pitta is the energy pattern of transformation or metabolism. Its distinguishing quality is the **hot,** and in excess it produces inflammation. So it's the Pitta energy pattern that creates the burning pelvic pain and burning on urination. Not surprisingly then, **cooling** postures reduce heat in the body:

<u>Moon salutation</u>

<u>Twists such as ardha matsyendrasana</u>

<u>Lying spinal twist jathara parivartanasana</u>

Hip opener (e.g., pigeon)

Other cooling poses include virabhadrasana 3, utkatanasana, navasana, and trikonsana.

All backward bends that stetch the areas of the solar plexus, navel, and abdominal area including the liver, spleen, stomach, small intestine, and heart are excellent for reducing Pitta.

Inversions in general are heating and should be avoided. Shoulder stand is **cooling**, but headstand is heating.

Yoga Postures for Kapha

Kapha's energy pattern is that of stability, and due to that it has a tendency to inertia. So instead of a slow sun salutation, the flow sequence would be done much more actively:

Sun salutation done vigorously

Backward bends: ustrasana or camel, setu bhandasana or bridge, hand knee or cat dog.

Side openers: parivritta parsvakonasana.

Oleation

I mentioned ghee as an excellent oil to use because it deals with the **dry** and **rough** qualities of Vata internally. External oleation is also an excellent way to deliver herbs to the body (the skin is the largest digestive surface of the body) through absorption and at the same time deal with the aging of skin, which becomes **dry** and **rough**.

Since the Vata energy pattern is responsible for the urgency and frequency of urination, the use of oil massage is highly therapeutic, with focus to **slow** application to the thighs and lower back and pelvis.

The beauty of self-applied oil massage is that you direct your attention to personalized areas, not just perform a generic massage. This is very valuable because it helps you find those areas that need attention the most. Only you know where it hurts because you are getting continual feedback from your body as to where to direct your attention.

Oleation for systemic disease takes advantage of the fact that the skin is the body's largest digestive surface. If the GI tract is not functioning well, the skin can provide a way by which herbs can be delivered to the body. In this way oleation becomes a means to treat systemic disease.

The use of mahanarayan oil for those with fibromyalgia can be extremely valuable due to Vata and its qualities being localized to specific areas of the body.

Marma and Therapeutic Oleation

As mentioned earlier, the use of castor oil packs fulfills many different energy science therapeutics at the same time. The bladder acupuncture or marma point is in the midline just above the pubic bone. Using castor as a **cool**ing herb in the pack reduces the **hot** quality from this energy focal point called marma.

The application of heat to the pack can serve as a muscle relaxant to the tense muscles of the lower abdomen, providing another therapeutic tool. Lastly the use of a **cool**ing aroma to the bladder marma point can make such a pack to the area very healing. **Cool**ing herbs such as mint, khus, sandalwood, jasmine, and rose can all be used. Essential oils come from the plant flowers and foliage. Attars are made from a sandalwood base with the accompanying essence, hence making it doubly therapeutic for IC treatment packs.

There are other points on the body that affect the bladder as well. Ani marma is one such point. It is located on the inside of the elbow on either side at the crease of the joint. This marma tonifies the bladder and treats bladder dysfunction. It also stimulates digestive strength and pancreatic function. Locally applying pressure with or without an essential oil can be useful when lying with your castor pack during an acute flare.

Oleation done with herbs can change thinking and hence healing. Herbs affect the mind, so they help direct healing by aiding in **subtle** decisions made around healing. For example, the choice arises out of nowhere about the use of marma points when doing oil massage, and you automatically begin using marma therapy as part of the routine.

Chapter Summary

Exercise improves metabolic fire and health, but overdoing is a Pitta thing to do and can be counterproductive in that it aggravates an already aggravated inflammatory energy pattern.

For IC patients, the best exercise is calming and cooling, reducing the **hot** and **mobile** qualities. External oleation can be highly therapeutic for Vata provocation, especially those with a fibromyalgia component. The use of herbs with oleation can improve decision making in healing.

The **hot** quality can be dissipated by breath exercises and yoga postures. Oleation with herbs and aromas can be therapeutic.

Epilogue: Life after IC

Disease of any kind is a wake-up call. It is in actuality a self-correcting process that shows us our imbalances.

You get a new body every year. Every cell has been recycled in that time frame, since the body undergoes perpetual, ongoing renewal. So it becomes a computer printout of your past year's choices, balancing, imbalancing, or both.

In other words, you are not doomed by your choices of the past. There's always hope for a new beginning because your DNA is always shape-shifting and changing due to the qualities that are being taken.

The sticking point for many with IC is that there comes a point when the flare symptoms are controlled and life is tolerable and manageable. Hydrodistention and fulguration, pharmaceuticals, alternative therapies, or most often combinations of all of the preceding play a role in diminishment in symptoms. But it all falls short of what you're looking for, which is complete cessation of IC.

Why bother? From an energy science view, the nagging imbalances are still present, just in reduced degree. These kinds of states can usher in new diseases that can become problematic. This new view of what it means to be healthy creates a new paradigm around the concept of health that is not held by our current matter science system of healing.

Then what happens when you heal IC and its sister diseases? What is in store for you then? Since there is no energy drain which occurs from any chronic disease, you can become more available to all your relationships with yourself and others. And when minor imbalances occur you have the tools to easily self correct.

You sleep better and feel better overall, with more mental clarity. You are able to focus your attention on matters of relevance, make good decisions, and experience good memory. You'll feel courage,confidence, cheerfulness, and contentment. You'll see your life with renewed enthusiasm .

I believe that health as you will know it will blossom into more and more revelations, making a time when each day is healthier than the next.

Health becomes a priceless journey that allows you to overcome your past and enjoy life in untold ways.

Good luck on your journey!

Appendix

Energy Makeup Questionnaire

When doing this energy assessment, we can see more than one response for each row. For example, in the line item Frame, a Pitta/Vata might respond to a medium symmetrical build, but also consider a thin lanky frame as also appropriate. In that case we would mark both Vata and Pitta columns. It would be highly unlikely that there be a circumstance where all three energy patterns would be selected. For example, it would be difficult to envision a situation where a mindbody would have **dry rough** thin skin under Vata, warm reddish in color and prone to irritation under Pitta and at the same time have thick moist smooth skin under Kapha. At times we may have trouble in deciding whether we have certain listed characteristics. In that case we might ask a spouse or friend who knows us well about responses particularly around temperament and under stress.

After we have totaled the numbers in the columns, the next step is to find out which are the two highest scores. For example, the Pitta column has 8 and Vata has 7 and Kapha has 4, it is clear that the mindbody energy constitution is Pitta/Vata(P/V)

	Vata	Pitta	Kapha
FRAME	I am thin, lanky, and slender with prominent joints and thin muscles.	I have a medium, symmetrical build with good muscle development.	I have a large, stocky or round build. My frame is broad, stout or thick.
WEIGHT	Low: I may forget to eat or have a tendency to lose weight.	Moderate: it is easy for me to gain or lose weight if I put my mind to it.	Heavy: I gain weight easily and have difficulty losing it.
EYES	My eyes are small and active.	I have a penetrating gaze.	I have large pleasant eyes.
COMPLEXION	My skin is dry, rough or thin.	My skin is warm, reddish in color and prone to irritation.	My skin is, thick, moist and smooth.

© Reprinted with permission from *Ayurevic Cooking for Self-Healing* by Dr. Vasant & Usha Lad

	Vata	Pitta	Kapha
HAIR	My hair is dry, brittle or frizzy.	My hair is fine with a tendency towards early thinning or graying	I have abundant, thick and oily hair
JOINTS	My joints are thin and prominent and have a tendency to crack.	My joints are loose and flexible.	My joints are large, well-knit and padded.
SLEEP PATTERN	I am a light sleeper with a tendency to awaken easily.	I am a moderately sound sleeper, usually needing less than eight hours to feel rested.	My sleep is deep and long. I tend to awaken slowly in the morning.
BODY TEMPERA-TURE	My hands and feet are usually cold and I prefer warm environments.	I am usually warm (regardless of the season) and prefer cooler environments.	I am adaptable to most temperatures but do not like cold, wet days.
TEMPERAMENT	I am lively and enthusiastic by nature. I like change.	I am purposeful and intense. I like to convince.	I am easy going and accepting. I like to be supportive.
UNDER STRESS	I become anxious and/or worried.	I become irritable and/or aggressive.	I become withdrawn and/or reclusive.
TOTAL* (total each column)			

* one point for each affirmative response; more than one point per row is appropriate

Food Guidelines for

Pitta/Vata

Anti-Inflammatory, Antidegenerative

	NO	MODERATION (Every 3-4 days)	YES
FRUITS	*Generally most dried fruit* Apples (raw) Cranberries Persimmons	*Generally most sour fruit* Apples (sour) Apricots (sour) Bananas Berries (sour) Cherries (sour) Dates (dry) Figs (dry) Grapes (green) Grapefruit Kiwi Lemons Limes Mangoes (green) Oranges (sour) Papaya Peaches Pears Pineapple (sour) Plums (sour) Pomegranates Prunes (dry) Raisins (dry) Rhubarb Strawberries Tamarind Watermelon	*Generally most sweet fruit* Apples (cooked and/or sweet) Applesauce Apricots (sweet) Avocado Berries (sweet) Cherries (sweet) Coconut Dates (fresh) Figs (fresh) Grapes (red and purple) Mangos (ripe) Melons Oranges (sweet) Pineapple (sweet) Plums (sweet) Prunes (soaked) Raisins (soaked)

© Reprinted with permission from *Ayurevic Cooking for Self-Healing* by Dr. Vasant & Usha Lad

	NO	MODERATION (Every 3-4 days)	YES
VEGETABLES	*Generally frozen, raw, dried, or pungent* Beet greens Burdock root Cabbage (raw) Cauliflower (raw) Corn Eggplant Horseradish Kohlrabi Olives, green Onions (raw) Peppers (hot) Prickly pear (fruit) Radish (raw) Tomatoes Turnips	Artichoke Beets (raw) Bitter melon Broccoli Brussel sprouts Cabbage Carrots (raw) Cauliflower (cooked) Celery Daikon radish Dandelion greens Garlic Green chilies Jerusalem artichoke Kale Leafy greens Leeks Lettuce Mushrooms Mustard greens Onions (cooked) Parsley Peas (raw)	*Generally sweet, bitter, or cooked* Asparagus Beets (cooked) Carrots (cooked) Cilantro Cucumber Fennel (anise) Green beans Leeks (cooked) Okra Olives, black Parsnips Peas (cooked) Potatoes, sweet Prickly Pear (leaves) Pumpkin Rutabaga Squash, Summer, Winter Taro root Zucchini

	NO	MODERATION (Every 3-4 days)	YES
VEGETABLES		Peppers (sweet) Potatoes, white Radishes (cooked) Spaghetti squash Spinach (cooked & raw) Sprouts (not spicy) Squash, winter Turnip greens Watercress Wheat grass sprouts	
GRAINS	Bread (with yeast) Buckwheat Cereal, cold, puffed Corn (including tortilla) Millet Muesli Oats (dry) Polenta Rye	Amaranth Barley Cereal (dry) Couscous Crackers Granola Oat bran Pasta Quinoa Rice (brown) Rice cakes Sago Spelt Tapioca Wheat bran	Durham flour Flatbreads (i.e., flour tortilla) Oats (cooked) Pancakes Rice (basmati, white, wild) Seitan (wheat meat) Sprouted wheat bread (Essene) Wheat
LEGUMES	Miso	Aduki beans Black beans Black-eyed peas Chick peas (garbanzo beans) Kidney beans	Mung beans Mung dal Split mung dal

© Reprinted with permission from *Ayurevic Cooking for Self-Healing* by Dr. Vasant & Usha Lad

	NO	MODERATION (Every 3-4 days)	YES
		Lentils (brown and red) Lima beans Navy beans Peas (dried) Pinto beans Soybeans Soy cheese Soy flour Soy milk Soy powder Soy sauce Soy sausage Split peas Tempeh Tofu Tur dal Urad dal White beans	
DAIRY	Cow's milk (powdered) Goat's milk (powdered) Yogurt (plain, frozen or w/ fruit)	Butter (salted) Buttermilk Cheese (hard) Ice cream Sour cream Yogurt (freshly made and diluted)	Butter (unsalted) Cheese (soft, not aged, unsalted) Cottage cheese Cow's milk Ghee Goats cheese (soft, unsalted) Goat's milk

	NO	MODERATION (Every 3-4 days)	YES
ANIMAL FOODS	Lamb Pork	Beef Chicken (white or dark) Duck Eggs with yolk Rabbit Salmon Sardines Seafood Tuna fish Turkey (white or dark) Venison	Buffalo Eggs (whites only) Fish (freshwater) Shrimp
CONDIMENTS	Chocolate Horseradish Salt (excess)	Black pepper Chili peppers Chutney, mango (spicy) Coriander leaves Dulse Gomasio Hijiki Kelp Ketchup Lemon Lime Lime pickles Mango pickles Mayonnaise Mustard Pickles Salt Scallions Seaweed Sprouts Tamari	Chutney, mango (sweet)

© Reprinted with permission from *Ayurevic Cooking for Self-Healing* by Dr. Vasant & Usha Lad

	NO	MODERATION (Every 3-4 days)	YES
		Soy sauce Vinegar	
NUTS		Almonds (with skin) Black Walnuts Brazil nuts Cashews Filberts Hazelnuts Macadamia nuts Peanuts Pecans Pine nuts Pistachios Walnuts	Almonds (soaked and peeled) Carole Coconut
SEEDS		Chia Popcorn (no salt, butter) Psyllium Pumpkin Sesame Tahini	Flax Halva Sunflower

	NO	MODERATION (Every 3-4 days)	YES
OILS	Corn	*For internal use* Almond Apricot Flaxseed Safflower Sesame Soy Sunflower	*For internal and external use:* (most suitable at top of list) Ghee Olive *For external use only* Coconut Avocado
BEVERAGES	Alcohol (hard) Caffeinated beverages Carbonated drinks Chocolate milk Coffee Cranberry juice Iced tea Icy-cold drinks Tomato juice V-8 juice *Herb Teas*: Basil Ginseng Mormon tea Red Zinger Yerba mate	Alcohol (beer, dry white, red and sweet wine) Apple juice, cider Black tea Carob Carrot juice Chai (hot spiced milk) Cool dairy drinks Grapefruit juice Lemonade Miso broth Mixed vegetable juice Orange juice Papaya juice Pear juice Pineapple juice Pomegranate juice Prune juice Sour juices Soy milk Vegetable bouillon	Almond milk Aloe vera juice or gel Apricot juice Berry juice (sweet) Cherry juice (sweet) Grain coffee Grape juice Mango juice Miso broth Peach nectar Rice milk *Herb Teas*: Bancha Chamomile Comfrey Fennel Ginger (fresh)

© Reprinted with permission from *Ayurevic Cooking for Self-Healing* by Dr. Vasant & Usha Lad

	NO	MODERATION (Every 3-4 days)	YES
		Herb Teas:	Lavender
		Ajwan	Lemon grass
		Alfalfa	Licorice
		Barley	Marshmallow
		Blackberry	Oat straw
		Borage	Peppermint
		Burdock	Sarsaparilla
		Catnip	Spearmint
		Chicory	
		Chrysanthemum	
		Cinnamon	
		Clove	
		Corn silk	
		Dandelion	
		Elder flower	
		Eucalyptus	
		Fenugreek	
		Ginger (dry)	
		Hawthorne	
		Hibiscus	
		Hops	
		Jasmine	
		Juniper berry	
		Kukicha	
		Lemon balm	
		Nettle	
		Orange peel	

	NO	MODERATION (Every 3-4 days)	YES
		Passion flower	
		Pennyroyal	
		Raspberry	
		Red clover	
		Rose hips	
		Saffron	
		Sage	
		Sassafras	
		Strawberry	
		Violet	
		Wintergreen	
		Yarrow	
SPICES		Ajwan	Basil (fresh)
		Allspice	Cinnamon
		Almond extract	Coriander
		Anise	Cumin
		Asafoetida (hing)	Dill
		Basil (dry)	Fennel
		Bay leaf	Ginger (fresh)
		Black pepper	Mint
		Caraway	Peppermint
		Cardamon	Saffron
		Cayenne	Spearmint
		Cloves	Turmeric
		Fenugreek	Wintergreen
		Garlic	
		Ginger (dry)	
		Mace	
		Marjoram	
		Mustard seeds	
		Neem leaves	

	NO	MODERATION (Every 3-4 days)	YES
		Nutmeg	
		Oranges peel	
		Oregano	
		Paprika	
		Parsley	
		Pippali	
		Poppy seeds	
		Rosemary	
		Sage	
		Salt	
		Savory	
		Star anise	
		Tarragon	
		Thyme	
		Vanilla	
SWEETENERS	White sugar	Honey (raw, unprocessed) Jaggery Maple syrup Molasses	Barley malt Fructose Fruit juice concentrates Rice syrup Sucanat Turbinado

	NO	MODERATION (Every 3-4 days)	YES
FOOD SUPPLEMENTS		Amino acids Barley green Bee pollen Brewer's yeast *Minerals:* Copper and Iron Royal jelly *Vitamins:* B2, B6, C, E, K, Bioflavonoids, and Folic acid	Aloe vera juice or gel *Minerals:* Calcium, Magnesium, and Zinc Spirolina Blue-green algae *Vitamins:* A, B1, B12, D, and E

© Reprinted with permission from *Ayurevic Cooking for Self-Healing* by Dr. Vasant & Usha Lad

Food Guidelines for

Pitta/Kapha

Anti-Inflammatory, Anticongestive

	NO	MODERATION (Every 4-5 days)	YES
FRUITS	*Generally most sour fruits* Apples (sour) Apricots (sour) Bananas Berries (sour) Cherries (sour) Grapefruit Grapes (green) Kiwi Oranges (sour) Pineapple (sour) Plums (sour) Rhubarb Tamarind	*Generally most sweet fruit* Avocado Coconut Cranberries Dates Figs (dry) Grapes (red and purple) Lemons Limes Mangos (ripe) Melons Oranges (sweet) Papaya Peaches Persimmons Pineapple (sweet) Plums (sweet) Strawberries Watermelon	Apples (sweet) Applesauce Apricots (sweet) Berries (sweet) Cherries (sweet) Pears Pomegranates Prunes Raisins

	NO	MODERATION (Every 4-5 days)	YES
VEGETABLES	Olives, green Tomatoes (raw)	*Generally most sweet vegetables* Beet greens Beets (raw) Burdock root Carrots (raw) Corn Cucumber Daikon radish Eggplant Garlic Green chilies Horseradish Kohlrabi Leeks (raw) Mustard greens Olives (black) Onions (raw) Peppers (hot) Potatoes, sweet Prickly pear (fruit) Pumpkin Radishes (raw) Spaghetti squash Spinach Squash, winter Taro root Tomatoes (cooked) Turnip greens Turnips Watercress	*Generally most bitter vegetables* Artichoke Asparagus Beets (cooked) Bitter melon Broccoli Brussel sprouts Cabbage Carrots (cooked) Cauliflower Celery Cilantro Dandelion greens Fennel (anise) Green beans Jerusalem artichoke Kale Leafy greens Leeks (cooked) Lettuce Mushrooms Okra Onions (cooked) Parsley Parsnip Peas Peppers, sweet Potatoes, white Prickly pear (leaves) Radishes (cooked)

© Reprinted with permission from *Ayurevic Cooking for Self-Healing* by Dr. Vasant & Usha Lad

	NO	MODERATION (Every 4-5 days)	YES
VEGETABLES		Zucchini	Rutabaga Sprouts (not spicy) Squash, summer Wheat grass sprouts
GRAINS	Bread (with yeast) Rice (brown)	Amaranth Buckwheat Corn Durham flour Millet Muesli Oats (dry/cooked) Pancakes Pasta Polenta Quinoa Rice (basmati, wild) Rice (white) Rice cakes Rye Spelt Wheat	Barley Cereal, dry, cold, or puffed Couscous Crackers Granola Oat bran Sago Seitan (wheat meat) Sprouted wheat bread (Essene) Tapioca Wheat bran
LEGUMES	Miso Soy sauce Urad dal	Mung beans Mung dal Kidney beans Soybeans Soy cheese Soy flour Soy powder	Aduki beans Black beans Black-eyed peas Chickpeas (garbanzo beans) Lentils, red and brown Lima beans

	NO	MODERATION (Every 4-5 days)	YES
		Soy sausage Tofu Tur dal	Navy beans Peas (dried) Pinto beans Soy milk Split peas Tempeh White beans
DAIRY	Butter (salted) Cheese (hard) Sour cream Yogurt (plain, frozen, or with fruit)	Butter (unsalted) Buttermilk Cheese (soft, not aged, and unsalted) Cottage cheese Cow's milk Ghee Goat's cheese (soft, unsalted, and not aged) Goat's milk, skim Ice cream Yogurt (freshly made and diluted)	Cottage cheese (from skimmed goat's milk)

© Reprinted with permission from *Ayurevic Cooking for Self-Healing* by Dr. Vasant & Usha Lad

	NO	MODERATION (Every 4-5 days)	YES
ANIMAL FOODS	Beef Chicken (dark) Duck Lamb Pork Salmon Sardines Seafood Tuna fish Turkey (dark)	Buffalo Eggs (with yolk) Shrimp	Chicken (white) Eggs (white only) Fish (freshwater) Rabbit Turkey (white) Venison
CONDIMENTS	Chocolate Gomasio Kelp Ketchup Lime pickle Mango pickle Mayonnaise Mustard (with vinegar) Pickles Salt Soy sauce Vinegar	Black pepper Chili peppers Chutney, mango, spicy Dulse Hijiki Horseradish Kombu Lemon Lime Mustard (without vinegar) Scallions Seaweed Tamari	Coriander leaves Sprouts
NUTS (including butters)	Almonds (with skins) Black walnuts Brazil nuts Cashews	Almonds (soaked and pealed) Coconut	Charole

	NO	MODERATION (Every 4-5 days)	YES
	Filberts Hazelnuts Macadamia nuts Peanuts Pecans Pine nuts Pistachios Walnuts		
SEEDS (including butters)	Sesame Tahini	Chia Flax Halva Popcorn (no salt, buttered) Psyllium Pumpkin Sunflower	Popcorn (no salt, butter)
OILS	*For internal and external use* Apricot Safflower *For internal use only:* Sesame	*For internal and external use* *Most suitable at top of list:* Corn Almond Olive Soy Flaxseed Primrose Walnut	*For internal and external use* *Most suitable at top of list in small amounts:* Sunflower Ghee Canola
		External use only: Avocado Coconut Sesame	

© Reprinted with permission from *Ayurvedic Cooking for Self-Healing* by Dr. Vasant & Usha Lad

	NO	MODERATION (Every 4-5 days)	YES
BEVERAGES	Alcohol (hard; sweet wine)	Alcohol (beer; red wine, dry white wine)	Aloe vera juice or gel
	Caffeinated beverages	Almond milk	Apricot juice
	Carbonated drinks	Apple cider	Berry juice (sweet)
	Cherry juice (sour)	Apple juice	Black tea (spiced)
	Chocolate milk	Berry juice (sour)	Carob
	Coffee	Carrot juice	Cherry juice (sweet)
	Grapefruit juice	Chai (hot, spiced milk)	Grain coffee
	Iced tea	Cherry juice (sour)	Grape juice
	Icy cold drinks	Cool dairy drinks	Mango juice
	Lemonade	Cranberry juice	Mixed vegetable juice
	Papaya juice	Miso broth	Peach nectar
	Sour juices	Orange juice (sweet)	Pear juice
	Tomato juice	Pineapple	Pomegranate juice
	V-8 juice	Rice milk	Prune juice
		Vegetable bouillon	Soy milk (hot and well spiced)
	Herb teas:		
	Red Zinger	*Herb teas:*	*Herb teas:*
	Rose hips	Ajwan	Alfalfa
		Basil	Bancha
		Borage	Barley
		Catnip	Blackberry
		Cinnamon	Burdock
		Clove	Chamomile
		Comfrey	Chicory
		Eucalyptus	Dandelion
		Fenugreek	Fennel
		Ginger (dry)	Ginger (fresh)
		Ginseng	Hibiscus
		Hawthorn	Jasmine
			Kukicha

	NO	MODERATION (Every 4-5 days)	YES
		Hops	Lavender
		Hyssop	Lemon balm
		Juniper berry	Lemon grass
		Licorice	Nettle
		Marshmallow	Passion flower
		Mormon tea	Peppermint
		Pennyroyal	Raspberry
		Sage	Red clover
		Sarsaparilla	Spearmint
		Sassafras	Strawberry
		Violet	Wintergreen
		Yerba mate	Yarrow
SPICES	Salt	Ajwan	Basil (fresh)
		Allspice	Cinnamon
		Almond extract	Coriander
		Anise	Cumin
		Asafoetida (hing)	Dill
		Basil (dry)	Ginger (fresh)
		Bay leaf	Mint
		Black pepper	Peppermint
		Caraway	Saffron
		Cardamom	Spearmint
		Cayenne	Turmeric
		Cloves	Wintergreen
		Fennel	
		Fenugreek	
		Garlic	

© Reprinted with permission from *Ayurvedic Cooking for Self-Healing* by Dr. Vasant & Usha Lad

	NO	MODERATION (Every 4-5 days)	YES
SPICES		Ginger (dry) Mace Marjoram Mustard seeds Neem leaves Nutmeg Orange peel Oregano Paprika Parsley Pippali Poppy seeds Rosemary Sage Savory Star anise Tarragon Thyme Vanilla	
SWEETENERS	Jaggery Molasses White sugar	Barley malt Fructose Honey (raw, not processed) Maple syrup Rice syrup Sucanat Turbinado	Fruit juice concentrates

	NO	MODERATION (Every 4-5 days)	YES
FOOD SUPPLEMENTS		Amino acids Bee pollen Royal jelly *Minerals*: Potassium, Copper, and Iron *Vitamins*: A, B1,B2, B6, B12, C, E, K, Bioflavanoids, Folic acid, and D	Aloe vera juice Barley green Brewer's yeast Spirolina Blue-green algae *Minerals*: Calcium, Magnesium, and Zinc

© Reprinted with permission from *Ayurvedic Cooking for Self-Healing* by Dr. Vasant & Usha Lad

Food Guidelines for

Vata/Kapha

Antidegenerative, Anticongestive

	NO	MODERATION (Every 4-5 days)	YES
FRUITS	*Generally most sour or dried fruits*	*Generally most sweet fruit*	Apples (cooked and/ or sweet)
	Apples (raw)	Avocado	Applesauce
	Apricots (sour)	Bananas	Apricots
	Berries (sour)	Coconut	Berries
	Cherries (sour)	Cranberries	Cherries
	Dates (dry)	Dates (fresh)	Grapes
	Oranges (sour)	Figs (dry or fresh)	Peaches
	Plums (sour)	Grapefruit	Pomegranates
	Prunes (dry)	Kiwi	Prunes (soaked)
	Raisins (dry)	Lemons	Raisins (soaked)
	Watermelon	Limes	Strawberries
		Mangoes	
		Melons	
		Oranges	
		Papaya	
		Pears	
		Persimmons	
		Pineapple	
		Plums	
		Pomegranates	
		Rhubarb	
		Tamarind	

	NO	MODERATION (Every 4-5 days)	YES
VEGETABLES	Olives, green Tomatoes (raw)	Artichoke Beet greens Bitter melon Broccoli Brussel sprouts Burdock root Cabbage (cooked) Carrots (raw) Cauliflower (cooked) Celery Corn (fresh) Cucumber Dandelion greens Eggplant Horseradish Jerusalem artichoke Kale Kohlrabi Leafy greens Lettuce Mushrooms Mustard greens Olives (black) Onions (raw) Parsnip Parsley Peas (cooked) Peppers (hot and sweet) Potatoes, white Potatoes, sweet Prickly pear (fruit and leaves) Pumpkin	*Generally most bitter vegetable and should be cooked* Asparagus Beets Carrots Cilantro Daikon radish Fennel (anise) Garlic Green beans Green chilies Leafy greens Leeks Okra Onions (cooked) Parsley Radishes (cooked) Rutabaga Squash, summer Turnip Watercress

© Reprinted with permission from *Ayurvedic Cooking for Self-Healing* by Dr. Vasant & Usha Lad

	NO	MODERATION (Every 4-5 days)	YES
VEGETABLES		Radishes (raw) Spaghetti squash Spinach Sprouts Squash, winter Taro root Tomatoes (cooked) Turnip greens Wheat grass sprouts Zucchini	
GRAINS	Bread (with yeast) Pasta Rice cakes Sago	Amaranth Barley Buckwheat Cereal (dry, cold, or puffed) Corn Couscous Crackers Durham flour Granola Millet Muesli Oats (dry/cooked) Oat bran Pancakes Polenta Quinoa Rice (brown, white) Rye Spelt Tapioca Wheat Wheat bran	Durham flour Quinoa Rice (basmati, wild) Seitan (wheat meat) Sprouted wheat bread (Essene)

	NO	MODERATION (Every 4-5 days)	YES
LEGUMES	Kidney beans Miso Soybeans Soy flour Soy powder Soy sauce	Aduki beans Black beans Black-eyed peas Chickpeas (garbanzo beans) Lentils (brown) Lima beans Navy beans Peas (dried) Pinto beans Kidney beans Soy cheese Split peas Tempeh Tofu (hot) Tur dal Urad dal White beans	Lentils (red) Soy milk Soy sausage Tur dal
DAIRY	Cheese (hard) Cow's milk (powdered) Goat's milk (powdered) Yogurt (plain, frozen,or with fruit)	Butter (unsalted) Buttermilk Cheese (soft, hard, not aged & unsalted) Cottage cheese (from cow's milk) Cheese (soft) Cow's milk Goat's milk Goat's cheese Ice cream Sour cream	Cottage cheese (from skimmed oat's milk) Ghee Goat's cheese (unsalted and not aged) Goat's milk (skim) Yogurt (diluted and spiced)

© Reprinted with permission from *Ayurvedic Cooking for Self-Healing* by Dr. Vasant & Usha Lad

	NO	MODERATION (Every 4-5 days)	YES
ANIMAL FOODS	Lamb Pork	Beef Buffalo Chicken (dark) Chicken (white) Duck Seafood Rabbit Salmon Sardines Tuna fish Turkey (dark) Turkey (white) Venison	Eggs Fish (freshwater) Shrimp
CONDIMENTS	Chocolate	Black pepper Chutney, mango, sweet Gomasio Horseradish Kelp Ketchup Kombu Lime Lime pickle Mango pickle Mayonnaise Pickles Salt Seaweed Soy sauce Vinegar Tamari	Chili peppers Chutney, mango, spicy Coriander leaves Dulse Hijiki Lemon Mustard (without vinegar) Scallions Seaweed Sprouts

	NO	MODERATION (Every 4-5 days)	YES
NUTS (including butters)	None	Almonds (soaked and pealed) Black walnuts Brazil nuts Cashews Coconut Filberts Hazelnuts Macadamia nuts Peanuts Pecans Pine nuts Pistachios Walnuts	Charole
SEEDS (including butters)	Psyllium	Flax Halva Popcorn (no salt, butter) Psylium Pumpkin Sesame Sunflower Tahini	Chia

© Reprinted with permission from *Ayurvedic Cooking for Self-Healing* by Dr. Vasant & Usha Lad

	NO	MODERATION (Every 4-5 days)	YES
BEVERAGES	Caffeinated beverages Carbonated drinks Cherry juice (sour) Chocolate milk Cold dairy drinks Coffee Iced tea Icy-cold drinks Soy milk (cold) Tomato juice V-8 juice Vegetable bouillon Herb teas: Red Zinger	Alcohol (beer, hard and dry and sweet white wine) Almond milk Apple juice Black Tea (spiced) Carob Chai (hot, spiced milk) Grapefruit juice Lemonade Miso broth Orange juice Papaya juice Pear juice Pineapple juice Pomegranate juice Prune juice Rice milk sour juice Herb teas: Alfalfa Barley Blackberry Burdock Catnip Chicory Cinnamon Cornsilk Crysanthemum Dandelion	Aloe vera juice or gel Apple cider Apricot juice Berry juice Carrot juice Cherry juice (sweet) Grain coffee Grape juice Mango juice Peach nectar Soy milk (hot and well spiced) Herb teas: Bancha Chamomile Chicory Clove Comfrey Fennel Fenugreek Ginger (fresh) Juniper berry Lavender Lemon grass Peppermint

	NO	MODERATION (Every 4-5 days)	YES
		Ginger (dry)	Sassafras
		Ginseng	Spearmint
		Hibiscus	Wintergreen
		Hops	
		Hyssop	
		Jasmine	
		Juniper berry	
		Kuchika	
		Lemon balm	
		Licorice	
		Marshmallow	
		Mormon tea	
		Nettle	
		Passion flower	
		Raspberry	
		Red clover	
		Rose hips	
		Sasaparilla	
		Strawberry	
		Violet	
		Yarrow	
		Yerba mate	
SPICES		Cayenne	Ajwan
		Fennel	Allspice
		Fenugreek	Almond extract
		Salt	Anise
		Vanilla	Asafoetida (hing)
			Basil
			Bay leaf
			Black pepper
			Caraway

	NO	MODERATION (Every 4-5 days)	YES
			Cardamom
			Cayenne
			Cinnamon
			Cloves
			Coriander
			Cumin
			Dill
			Garlic
			Ginger
			Mace
			Marjoram
			Mint
			Mustard seed
			Neem leaves
			Nutmeg
			Orange peel
			Oregano
			Paprika
			Parsley
			Peppermint
			Rosemary
			Saffron
			Sage
			Savory
			Spearmint
SWEETENERS	Jaggary Maple syrup Molasses White sugar	Barley malt Fructose Molasses Rice syrup Sucanat Turbinado	Fruit juice (concentrate) Honey (raw and not processed)

	NO	MODERATION (Every 4-5 days)	YES
FOOD SUPPLEMENTS		Barley green Brewers yeast *Minerals:* Potassium *Vitamins:* A, B1, B2, B12, C, D, and K	Aloe vera juice or gel Amino acids Bee pollen Blue-green algae Royal jelly Spirolina *Minerals:* Calcium, Magnesium, Copper, Iron & ZInc *Vitamins:* B6, E, Folic acid and Bioflavonoids

© Reprinted with permission from *Ayurvedic Cooking for Self-Healing* by Dr. Vasant & Usha Lad

Food Incompatibilities

(as important as NO list)

Don't Eat:	With
Beans	Fruit, cheese, eggs, fish, milk, meat, yogurt
Eggs	Fruit (especially melons), beans, cheese, fish, khichari, MILK, meat, yogurt
Fruit	NO other food Eaten alone except dates and milk
Grains	Fruit, tapioca
Honey**	With equal GHEE by weight (e.g., 1 tsp. honey with 3 tsp. ghee); boiled or cooked honey
Hot drinks	Mangos, cheese, fish, meat, starch, yogurt
Lemons	Cucumbers, milk, tomatoes, yogurt
Melons	EVERYTHING—especially dairy, eggs, fried food, grains, starches. Melons more than most fruit should be eaten alone or left alone.
Milk	BANANAS, cherries, melons, sour fruits, bread containing yeast, fish, kitchari, meat, yogurt
Nightshades	Dairy products, melon, cucumber
Radishes	Bananas, raisins, milk
Tapioca	Fruit BANANA MANGO, beans, raisins, jaggery
Yogurt	MILK, cheese, eggs, fruit, meat, fish, hot drinks, meat, nightshades

Foods in CAPITALS are the most difficult combinations.

*These guidelines are by no means an exhaustive list. It must be remembered that a proper Ayurvedic diet should also consider nutritional value, constitution, season, age, and any disease condition.

**According to ancient Ayurvedic literature, honey should never be cooked. If cooked, the molecules become a nonhomogenized glue that adheres to mucus membranes and clogs subtle channels, producing toxins. Uncooked honey is nectar. Cooked honey is considered poison.

Steps in Energy Science Nutrition

Any suggestion of lifestyle change can cause fear because it takes you out of your comfort zone and places you in the unknown. If you embark on a new nutritional behavior pattern, then questions arise that raise doubts as to whether this is such a good idea. But as a result of your fear of change, you stay stuck in the same well-worn ruts that keep you entrenched in poor health.

So the way out of your fears is to first recognize that you have them. Everyone who walks on this planet has fears, and we all have many ways of preventing us from seeing what these fears are. If you become familiar with your favorite coping strategies, you have made a huge step in confronting the resistance that inhibits you from making health-promoting changes in your life. When you promote lifestyle choices, you will bring about excellent energy, lightness in body, superior digestion, improved appetite, greater physical strength and stamina, stronger resistance to disease, and, most important, a sense of real happiness.

Suggestions

Choose those things that are easiest to do first.

Be patient with yourself and make baby steps in the direction of lifestyle change.

Stop self-criticism for not doing it right.

Carry nutritional information with you wherever you go for eight weeks to make a habit.

Understand the faith-trust cycle. If you have some faith that this lifestyle change will bring about a better feeling of well-being and go about doing some work, you experience feeling better. This brings about more trust in the process, which in turn promotes more faith. The process self-perpetuates itself.

Improving Digestion and Balance with All Six Tastes

Have you ever gotten up from eating a meal having consumed enough food but still feeling hungry? Energetically the reason for the lack of satiety or fullness after a meal is the lack of one or more of the six tastes. A meal will bring about satisfaction if all six tastes are provided. A churan, which means powder, is made of spices that provide the tastes of sweet, sour, salty, pungent, bitter, and astringent. So a meal of French fries with a churan, although not completely nutritious, is complete from an energetic perspective because all six tastes have been provided.

Sprinkling the following herbal combinations on prepared food or, better yet, including them in the cooking will ensure that the meal includes all six tastes.

Pitta/Vata	Pitta/Kapha — Vata/Kapha
Fennel seeds	Black pepper
Cardamom	Cinnamon
Cumin	Cumin
Coriander	Fenugreek
Turmeric	Turmeric
Sucanat	Sucanat
Mineral salt	Mineral salt

The amount of each of the herbs is left to individual taste. It may be surprising to you how satisfied you can feel when using these herbal combinations with your meals. These herbal combinations also serve as important digestants to stimulate the digestive enzyme system, which is especially important if the digestive fire is compromised by stagnant energy.

Another commercial churan, hingwastak, is a classical mixture and is readily available. Another simple recipe that we can use is:

Sweet 1 part sugar, Sucanat, or turbinado crystallized cane sugar

Sour 1 part lime or lemon juice

Salty pinch of rock salt

Pungent pinch of cayenne pepper

Bitter pinch of turmeric

Astringent ¼ tsp of fenugreek powder

Making Kitchari

Kitchari is a very simple meal to digest and because of that it improves the digestive strength or agni of the body. It is balancing as it offers all 6 tastes and is an excellent source of easily digestable protein. Due to its ease of digestion it is a way of giving your GI tract a day off like juice fasting.

It is very useful in cases where ama or stagnant energy is clinically present or when it is obvious on the tongue. Its most common usage is for preparatory cleansing, detoxification periods, as well as post cleansing.

However it can be used for regular daily consumption but it can be constipating. When used as regular daily nutrition, the variations are endless.

The basic recipe and its stages include:

Split yellow mung dal

Vegetables of choice based on your unique energy pattern as above

Basmati rice

Ghee

Spices: fennel seeds, black mustard seeds (optional), hing(asafetida), cumin, coriander, turmeric, and fresh ginger

Condiments: ghee, cilantro, unsweetened, coconut flakes, mineral salt, and lime

Stages

1 Cooking the dal Add 0.5 cup dal to 4 cups boiling water. As the preparation continues may need to add more water. Add more or less based on desired consistency, that is, more water soupy, less water more full bodied.

2 Add vegetables Chopped vegetables of choice **Anytime Anyone Veggies** asparagus carrots fennel green beans leeks okra parsnip peas rutabaga summer squash sweet potato

3 Spice Preparation In a separate small cast iron skillet melt 2 Tablespoons of ghee and to this heated **oil** add 0.5 teaspoon of fennel seeds, 0.5 teaspoon black mustard seeds (if Pitta is aggravated don't use), and allow to cook until popping. When the seeds are done, add a pinch of hing, 0.5 teaspoon each of powdered cumin, coriander, and turmeric. When the seeds and spices are blended and heated, add 2 Tablespoons of fresh chopped ginger root. The amounts of the spices can be increased in desired to make a bit of a paste. You can add more ghee if desired as well. **Offer this spice mixture to the cooking dal and vegetable mixture.**

4 Cooking phase Allow the mixture to simmer for 15 minutes to cook the spices together with the dal vegetable mix and the kitchari is done.

5 Basmati rice Cook the basmati separately and then serve the kitchari over the rice.

6 Addition of condiments   Ghee (V), chopped coconut (P), and cut cilantro leaf (VPK), fresh grated ginger (VPK), lime (VPK) can be added to the mixture. Mineral salt to taste.

Kitchari variations: White chicken breast to the cooking mixture can be added if you and/or your family desires meat this need can be met. Use of cashews or soaked and peeled almonds is another way to add variety. Of course the vegetable choices are limited to what is available in the market. Instead of using basmati rice, especially during the summer months, placing the kitchari mixture over baked potato (white or sweet) is another possibility. As discussed earlier, making a soup by adding lots more water can be quite nice.

If the kitchari seems too bland and is being used for regular meal preparation and not for cleansing, using mustard or other condiments for taste can be appealing.

Leftover kitchari: Leftovers kept in the refridgerator less than 48 hours maximum is safe and is sometimes necessary with a busy lifestyle. You can intentionally cook just the split mung and spices and save this mixture. In the next 24 hours you can steam vegetables of choice and add to the pre-prepared split mung mixture and serve over rice with condiments.

Making Ghee

Ghee is clarified butter and is free of harmful fatty acids due to its preparation. It is the oily essence of milk and is free of lactose, so those who feel they are allergic to lactose can use ghee without problems. If you have problems, it's not the ghee! Because it does not contain fatty acids, the shelf life is long. It does not require re-frigeration because there are no fats to become rancid.

Ghee, because of its **sharp/penetrating, dry, mobile, light,** and **subtle** qualities, is a truly a medicinal food and has the qualities of digestive fire.

It penetrates the tissue layers of the energy body quickly and can serve as a vehicle to carry herbs to the tissues. You can think of ghee as a medicinal taxicab. Your own preparation of ghee in the kitchen is simple. Four pounds of unsalted pure butter will make four pints of ghee. Butter has water as one of its components, so you can use this fact to help tell you when the butter has been cooked long enough to burn off the fatty acids in the butter.

After the butter is melted, a rich, fatty foam will accumulate over the surface of the cooking liquefied butter. As the cooking progresses, this foam layer—made up of fatty acids—gets less and less as the fatty acids are burned up by the heat of cooking. These fatty acids become a waxy, oily, gooey substance at the bottom of the cooking vessel as the process of ghee formation takes place.

You know when you have burned off the fatty acids from the butter when the water content is gone. The bubbling that occurs throughout cooking begins to subside and the liquid becomes quiet, although the bubbling doesn't go away completely. (If you leave the butter cooking for any longer, the fatty acids at the bottom of the vessel will burn and impart a brown color to the liquid ghee.) The ghee is then strained through cheesecloth to keep the burned-off fatty acids from contaminating the ghee, which should be placed into glass storage containers.

The final product should have a nutty aroma and a rich yellow color in its liquid state and be translucent enough that you can see through the glass jar. In its solid state, ghee should be soft, light yellow, and easily spreadable. When heat is applied, it melts quickly.

Meditation

A quiet mind is your servant; a turbulent mind is your enemy."

As more balance is achieved through the physical work described in this book the more the mind will become settled. A quiet mind is an expression of balance. Meditation is also a way to help reduce mental turbulence and is regarded as a health activity not a religious activity. Prayer is important but it should not be confused with meditation.

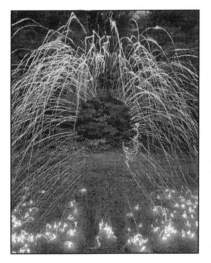

There are two reasons to meditate. Meditation is a tool to quiet the mind. Often you think the mind is quiet but at the deeper subconscious levels of the thinking process there can be a great deal of turbulence. Due to unprocessed subconscious thoughts, feelings, and emotions, mental activity can be so distracting and so lively that it causes anxiety and physiologic turmoil.

The second reason to meditate is to find out who you really are. You are not your thoughts but you are the observer of the thoughts. Through meditation you get more in touch with that observer who over time becomes more prominent than the busy mind.

There are many misconceptions about meditation including that the practice should be austere and disciplined. Meditation is play and is not serious. Nothing in Nature is serious except humans. The outer trappings are unimportant (special clothes or things to sit on, physical sensations such as candles, aromas, music).

When we exercise the physical body we are doing something with our bodies. However the best thing to do for ourselves is to quiet the mind which is in fact quieting the body as well. The best description of the inner experience of meditation is that I am simply not doing.

The practice advocated for people beginning practice is breath awareness. This technique uses the breath as the vehicle to quiet the mind's internal dialogue. Just watch the breath come in and go out. If you like you can add a verbal cue, *So* on inhalation and *Ham* on exhalation. These sounds mimic the sound of the breath on inhalation and exhalation. When distracted by thoughts simply bring your attention back to the breath and *So Ham* (a mantra which means instrument of the mind).

There are no strict rules about meditation but guidelines are useful.

Guidelines for Meditation

Bracket the day's activities with the practice.

Aim for twenty minutes in the morning and twenty minutes in the evening.

Regularity of practice is key to derving benefits. Regular time spent is more important than the amount of tme spent, that is, five minutes is better than not doing it at all.

The only difference between daydreaming and meditation is that in meditation you choose the breath or mantra when distracted by thoughts when you realize you are involved in thinking

Look for a consistent place to practice.

Maintain an upright posture. Practice alertness. You can lie down but this often suggests to the body that you want to sleep so it is better to be upright.

Exercise and eat after the practice.

Meditate one to two hours before bedtime as you may be too alert if meditating at bedtime and have trouble falling asleep.

Remember not to judge the meditation such that one session is better or worse than another. There is no right or wrong meditation. The busier meditations may be releasing lots of pent up energy.

There can only be three experiences during meditation.

A Fall asleep and this means you need more sleep

B Have lots of thoughts. This is normal and a release of pockets of energy that need to be released. The types of thoughts that occur are meaningless.

C Experience silence or fully awake without thoughts. This is also called "slipping into the gap" (the gap is the space between thoughts which is widened with meditation). It is an aler t state of awareness of silence devoid of thoughts. This is not the "goal" in meditation. Meditation is a process without goals or end results.

How do you know whether meditation is worthwhile?

Did my mind find the silence I was seeking?

Was I psychologically comfortable during and after the session?

Did my old self change as a result of having meditated?

Did my life become more meaningful?

Did my life become richer and fuller?

Is there more truth in my existence?

Have I stopped worrying about things?

Am I seeing meaningful coincidences?

Online Resource

Interstitial Cytitis Association, last modified May 7, 2013, accessed May 3, 2013, http://www.ichelp.com/Interstitial Cytitis Network, last modified May 7, 2013, accessed May 13, 2012, http://www.ic-network.com/

National Ayurvedic Medical Association, last modified May 15, 2013, accessed May 20, 2103, http://www.ayurvedanama.org/

Energy science blog, modified weekly, accessed weekly, http://www.drbilldean.com/

Energy science website, modified every six months, accessed weekly, http://www.foodsheal.com/

IC website, modified weekly, accessed weekly, http://www. Icdiet.com/

IC blog, modified weekly, accessed weekly, http://www. ic-solutions.tv/

Benefits of meditation, http://bit.ly/mfsZc1, MIT study, May 2011

About the Author

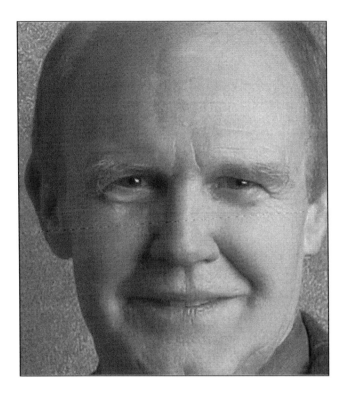

Dr Bill Dean began practicing urology in 1979 and retired from practice in 2011 to begin an alternative medicine fellowship at the Ayurvedic Institute in Albuquerque, New Mexico.

Due to his training, Dr Bill is uniquely positioned to serve as your guide to compare and contrast the matter and energy science healing disciplines. "When the current allopathic or matter science healing approach doesn't have an answer, the energy science discipline of Ayurveda can certainly shed light and help with difficult clinical problems," says Dr Bill. "This is because of how the two models differ in how they do their healing."

Dr. Bill became interested in the alternative medical discipline of Ayurveda through the Chopra organization in 1995. This introduction showed him the science behind the discipline that was grounded in modern physics.

In 2000, having his own medical problems, he sought help at the Ayurvedic Institute and over the years has watched his health gradually but dramatically improve. He realized that going to work, eating, sleeping, and communicating in relationships did not translate into health, and that we often do not realize how sick we are. As he began doing this healing slowly over the years, problems such as chronic edema from varicose veins cleared, longstanding bowel issues with poor digestion gradually resolved with resultant improved bone density, longstanding skin lesions cleared, and a healthy understanding of relationships improved.

He saw that real healing took time, and through the experience he realized tools and techniques that could be used to reverse the disease process. Dr. Bill began seeing healing in a more complete way. This improvement in his health brought enthusiasm to use some simple therapies in his urology practice for IC, since there were no consistently good results with standard therapies in urology.

Dr. Bill slowly began to realize that the medical matter science healing tradition that he was practicing was a disease detection and treatment program. Yes, it could provide semi-emergent treatments for concerning conditions such as cancer, but there were no means to treat chronic disease and certainly no system of prevention using this system of healing.

In contrast, he found that the science of Ayurveda used a different model of healing, not one founded on molecular expressions of disease but on physiologic energetic imbalances in the mindbody. In 2004 he wrote a paper on the results of a study showing the improvement of men, women, and children using Ayurvedic nutrition and aloe vera gel. The results are reported at icdiet.com. In six weeks, 91 percent of the patients had a 50 percent reduction in symptoms. This was indeed exciting and energized Dr. Bill to continue expanding on this approach to healing. He presented this paper at the Northwest Urological Society annual meeting in Vancouver, British Columbia, Canada, in 2005.

With continued success using Ayurvedic principles in the office, he began actively blogging at drbilldean.com, which began contrasting the matter science or molecular healing approach that he was practicing with that of the Ayurvedic or energy science approach. In the ensuing years of practice, he continued to help his patients' pain with what he now calls an energy science of healing. This led to the 2010 publication of *Foods Heal: Why Certain Foods Help YOU Feel Your Best,* which uses the nutritional model to show the differences between the current matter science medical discipline and the Ayurvedic or the energy science medical discipline.

Says Dr. Bill: "Most chronic debilitating diseases are not adequately managed, since the molecular model does not understand the origins of disease. The energy science medical model shows how imbalances created in the energy field percolate up and manifest into the matter field in a very distant time frame. This is the key to healing these debilitating conditions."

So Dr. Bill wants to show people who come to him how this energy science of Ayurveda can heal the chronic disease of IC. "That's a tall order," he says, "but with my past experience and what I have learned during my fellowship, it is definitely possible if IC sufferers want to take on the challenge." He actively blogs about using energy science aspects of IC at ic-solutions.tv.

Dr. Bill is married and has three children and five grandchildren He graduated from the University of Nebraska's medical school in 1972 and has done fellowships in nephrology and pediatric urology and just completed the year in alternative medicine at the Ayurvedic Institute. He enjoys skiing, backpacking, and staying physically fit through daily exercise.

Other Books by Dr. Bill Dean

Foods Heal: Why Certain Foods Help YOU Feel Your Best

June 2010

Publisher: CreateSpace

Available in Kindle Store

Contrasts the current molecular science of healing with that of the energy science using nutrition.

IC Bladder Syndrome Kindle book series

Interstitial Cystitis Bladder Syndrome: The Role of the Gut in GERD and IBS

Interstitial Cystitis Bladder Syndrome: Fibromyalgia

Interstitial Cystitis Bladder Syndrome: Chronic Prostatitis

Legal Disclaimer

The information contained in this book should not be considered medical advice. If you have been given the diagnosis of interstitial cystitis, you should have a urological evaluation.

The purpose of this book is to educate. The author and publisher shall have neither liability nor responsibility to any person or entity with respect to any loss, damage, or injury caused or alleged to be caused directly or indirectly by the information in this book.

Metabalance

5299 Olympic Dr NW

Gig Harbor, WA 98335 USA

Made in the USA
Las Vegas, NV
01 April 2022

46661971R00109